A Funny Thing Happened

Carl W. Otte

Phoenix, AZ

Dedicated to Retired USAF Lt Co Bob Cooley
1932–2016

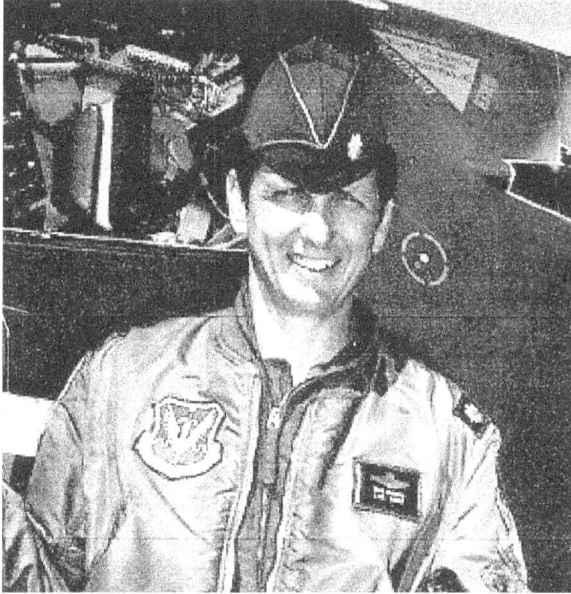

Robert Cooley was a friend and neighbor of mine for the last sixteen years of his life. He was a native Phoenician and a true American hero. His fighter plane was shot down on the outskirts of Hanoi and he was rescued by helicopter. Bob named my book by saying "Why don't you just call it 'A Funny Thing Happened'"?

CONTENTS

Preface

The title of this book shall be *A Funny Thing Happened*. It will be classified as a book of fiction, simply because I don't want to do the research to prove every nitpicking point. It will, however, be based upon either my own memory of events or as others have told them. My intent is for it to be mostly entertaining and a little informative. The idea of the book was, originally, to relay all the good emergency medicine stories. After starting the writing, though, I realized that life in general had many good events, such as growing up on a farm and raising four girls, so I have expanded the timeframe to encompass my lifetime. I want all animal lovers to know that no animals were injured in these episodes, only humans.

Acknowledgments

Many thanks to my wife Twyla and my daughters Kimberly, Valerie, Pamela, and Patricia for their contributions to the events in our lives and for their gentle guidance. My sisters Irma, Vera, and Ruth have also added their remembrances of times past. Maximum credit goes to Diana Grabau of Seize the Day Edits for turning this from an amateur to a professional document.

CHAPTER ONE

Inception

This is an accumulation of stories and happenings that have occurred during my nearly eighty-two years. My intention is to record mostly the humorous or interesting happenings. My memories of what took place during certain time frames is the absolute truth as I remember it. A few times, I have relayed stories told to me, and in those cases I have identified that. Some of the family information has been relayed to me and I have recorded it.

***

I was born in September of 1936, and my folks had been married for about one year prior. This placed their marriage and my birth at the end of The Great Depression. That fact alone greatly affected the way we were brought up and the values we were taught. I say we, because three more sisters (Irma, Vera, and Ruth) followed within the next eight years.

Times were tough and money short in those first years of my parents' married life. Farm and bank records show that the folks had to occasionally borrow money from Grandpa Otte for even relatively minor items. The records show that the loans were always paid back. At one time, Dad had an account in a bank in Yorktown, Iowa (a small town of about eighty-five people now). Martha, my mother, graduated from high school and worked as a teller at one of the banks in Clarinda before the marriage.

A story has circulated that mother was attacked by one of the town's men on the way home from work and that she hurt him badly. It occurred in front of the old library. The good-old-boy system still prevailed then, so I don't believe anything ever came of this, except that one of the town fathers sported some painful bruises for a while. Dad was always so proud at how fast Mother could count coins. We believe that Dad had little if any high school and then had to stay home to help farm. Dad said jokingly that he went through high school—in the east door and out the west.

Education was not thought to be important to the German farmers of that time. My folks were a very religious and moral couple. Religion, farming, church, and raising a good family were their life. The folks loved to have company, or what we would call entertaining, and they had the large home, as shown on the book cover, with a screened-in porch to accommodate guests. It appears that the Muellers (Mother's family) gathered at our place about once per month.

These gatherings would include Paul and Edna Mueller, Carl and Ada Mueller, Eddie and Tina Mueller, and Mother's sister Wilma and her husband George Redmon. The men always found something to argue over, and each thought they had won. They picked on Uncle George mercilessly, and he had to take a lot of antacids. Wilma and George seemed to always be out of cigarettes and spent much of their time looking for them. They must have bought only one pack at a time, so they had to go to town often to get some "cigs."

Any relatives who were in the area would spend at least some time at the Otte farm and would be fed royally. A large baked ham or fried chicken, potatoes and gravy, several vegetables, and bread and dessert were standard fare. Beer and other drinks were always available. I know now that the folks really could not afford all that company and food. Ladies did pitch in, at that time, to help with preparation—but most of the work fell to Mother. We seldom ate out, because we could not afford that. Always very hospitable to guests in their house, the folks passed that gene on, I believe. They were so proud of the house, farm, and crops. Several farm ponds (one was about two acres in size with an island) provided hours of fishing, hunting, and ice-skating pleasures for us and friends. Dad felt sure that everyone would want to use those ponds and was so proud when they did.

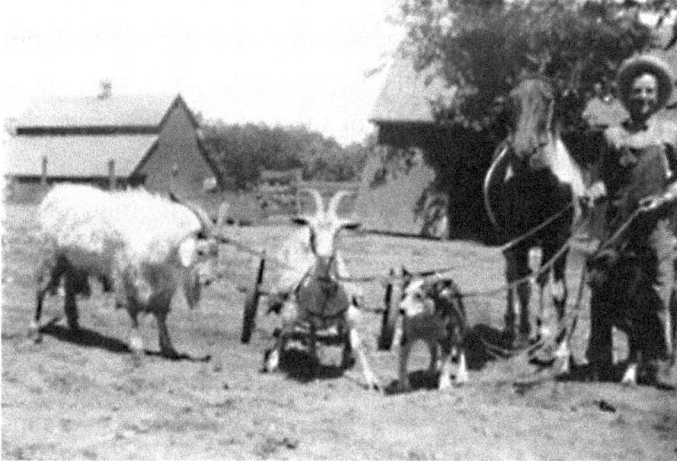

My dad showing early farming. It looks pretty miserable. I don't think he did this as a joke. All the men were quite thin at that time, probably from all the hard work.

I am getting ahead of myself. I want to talk about the grandparents. Grandfather Charlie and Grandmother Minnie Otte (my dad's parents) were salt-of-the-earth people who would never hurt anybody. I don't know much about my great grandfather, Charlie's dad, except that he died when Grandpa was twelve years old. I assume that either he or Grandpa built up the Otte homeplace. Grandpa must not have finished grade school, as he needed to take over the farm at age twelve. Maybe that is why he retired to town and off the farm when Dad got married. Grandpa had to be in his forties at that time.

I know nothing of my great grandmother on my grandmother Minnie's side, but she was a Goecker. I believe that the Otte grandparents gave Dad the home place, which sat about six miles northwest of Clarinda, Iowa, and they bought Dad's older brother John 160 acres south of Yorktown. Whether this arrangement caused friction, I'm not sure. I have heard that these farms were not totally free of debt, so there would have been some mortgages passed along with these gifts.

Farmers in the late 1800s and early 1900s seemed to do well and could give farms to their kids. Grandpa Otte (Charlie) seemed to be quite progressive for his time. He had a windmill that produced electricity which was stored in a large battery bank, located on shelves over the stairs to the basement of the house. That electrical system was eighty years ahead of its time, and there has been some editorial interest lately in that windmill/battery system. Unfortunately, there is nothing of his hardware left.

Their house was two stories plus a basement. They had a deep cave which served as a cool place for fruit and potato storage, and it also functioned as the neighborhood storm cellar. The cave provided cooling for the homemade beer and wine as well. The temperature seemed quite constant. I'd guess around sixty degrees. No wonder neighbors liked to come there for "storm parties."

The homeplace where my sisters and I grew up must have been quite a spectacular farm place in its time during the late 1800s through about 1980. That time period would have covered my great grandfather's, my grandfather's, and my father's lives. Things began to fall apart when it came to my generation, and there were no children to handle the farm operations. The land itself was well cared for and actually improved considerably during the 1980-2000 timeframe when Larry Sunderman farmed the land for the four children of Orval and Martha.

The farm buildings and 3.14 acres were sold off soon after Dad's death, and that was the beginning of the decline in the homeplace buildings. The house was lived in only occasionally after it had new owners, and it declined rapidly. The entire two-hundred-acre farm was sold to Doyle and Donna Wagoner and his son Zachary, very good farmers who lived across the road, around the year 2000. He has since purchased the 3.14 acres with the buildings on it but had to bulldoze the house because it became unsafe.

Doyle has been very good to allow our family access to the buildings for sentimental reasons. He found a black sign in a pile of boards that said "Accordions" and "Music," which came from my studio in the 1950s. He gave it to my sisters, knowing that it might be of sentimental value to me. These boards are now on the wall of our garage. Doyle has also been careful to preserve a patch of perennial sweet peas along a fence near where the old garden would have been. I had started those around 1950, and they are a beautiful light purple color. Pam carried flowers from those plants in her wedding, and we frequently see table centerpieces of those blooms when we are at Vera's for meals.

The rest of the buildings at the homeplace included two barns, a tool shed, a hog house, a granary, and a garage. The garage was a large building that would easily hold up to four vehicles, plus a large area like a blacksmith shop, its own stove, and a separate back room. The building had been one of the original school buildings for Immanuel Church and it had "1869" framed above the garage door— which must have been when it was built. Grandpa Otte had bought the building from the church sometime in the early 1900s and had moved it three-and-a-half miles, from the church area to his home. The move must have been quite an event, because Mervil (Twyla's dad) and others have talked of it. The building was pulled, intact, either on logs or a wheel mechanism with the power being provided by an early steam engine.

The building was quite solid and made a great shop and shed. It had its own heating system—a potbelly stove—and I remember placing straw bales in a circle on the floor for neighborhood telephone meetings. We had eight families on our party line, and during these meetings we conducted business related to running the phone system.

On the back wall of the large room sat a pump organ with all the stops, which I can remember playing. It was probably moved with the school, and I wish we had kept it. The blackboards were still in place on the west wall, along with chalk and erasers. Nails or pegs stuck outward from one-foot boards all the way around the room near the ceiling. The best corn ears were hung from the nails to dry and were then used as seed corn the next year, before the advent of hybrid seed corn. The garage was only one of several well-built buildings on the place, and it burned down, unfortunately, under the ownership of the first family who bought the four acres. The corncrib, just east of the house, was another good building, and I know it was built by Grandpa and Grandma Otte, as we found their names inscribed in the cement, along with dates. The building must have been the cat's meow when built. It had a strong electric elevator which took the ear corn up and dumped it into one of the three slatted bins for drying.

Grandpa was known as a hard worker, although I never witnessed that. He was good at witching for water. He retired to Clarinda about one year before I was born and had been farming about thirty-five years by that time. He did come out to the farms often to help his two married boys.

I have often wondered lately just what Grandpa and Grandma Otte lived on in their forty years of retirement. They had no investments that I know of, and no Social Security until late in their lives. They did own eight acres on the west edge of Clarinda on Highway 2. A large house in which they lived sat on the property, as well as a cute, smaller house, which they rented out. They had a large garden and a few milk cows and processed a large amount of honey in their basement. I'm sure their needs were few, and they seldom traveled. Their home was always welcoming, and I spent considerable time there in the summers.

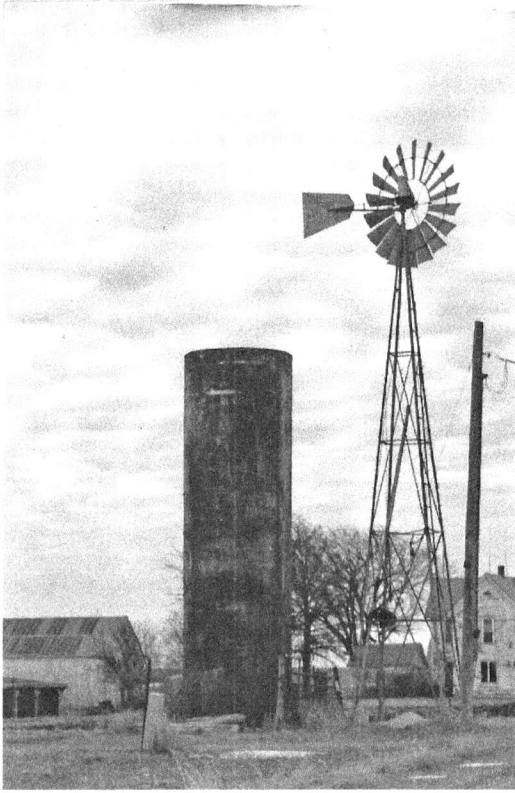

The windmill and water tower still stand just to the west of the home place. The buildings are mostly burned or buried and the area is farmed. The Wagoners, who bought the farm, have built a nice home just to the left of this picture. The location at the top of the hill is a much better, safer location for a house. Older photos would have shown another windmill just to the east beyond the house for supplying the water, as well as the electricity for the battery system mentioned in the book.

The small house was rented to the Gregorys. They had a boy who was a little younger than I was, and we played together a lot. He had a pet pigeon in the house, which I thought was great fun. There was a neighbor we did not like who lived east of the big house. Donald and I threw dirt clods we got from Grandma's garden at the west side of his newly painted house. He did not like us any better after that. Grandpa often threatened to spank us with his razor strap, but I don't remember that he ever needed to. We thought that would hurt like the dickens.

Grandma's mother (Bredehorst) died when I was in preschool. I remember exactly where the casket was placed in Grandma's living room, and I was coaxed to kiss or touch the departed, which I did not like one bit. The home, built mostly of stone and cement, still stands today. I don't know whether Grandpa is the one who built it.

Grandparents Otte bought eighty acres of land about three miles west of Clarinda when they were about sixty-five years old. They moved there from Clarinda and built a totally new small farm, much of it with their own hands. They had a new house along with several farm buildings, with large gardens and flower patches of roses and petunias. They canned huge amounts of their produce, and a visit there always included a tour of the fruit cellar, along with samples to take home. Grandpa planted several acres of fruit trees on the hills behind the house, along with large strawberry patches and raspberries. By that age, they were very much following the traditions that had been passed down to them, and they disapproved of the signs of progress. It seemed that they always planted too much.

Grandpa Charlie (Carl) and Minnie still spoke German some of the time. The mealtime prayer was short: "Abba Liba Fater, Amen." Grandma's house always smelled like freshly baked bread or bacon and eggs. Grandma remembered that, during her childhood, Indians passed by on their trail behind her homeplace, which was the Otto Goecker home several miles west of our homeplace. Grandma was the kindest person that you could imagine and spent her life in concern for others and taking care of Grandpa. And Grandpa talked of taking his turn protecting the German Lutheran Church in Yorktown with firearms, probably during World War I.

Grandma died from pancreatic cancer on the day our twins Pat and Pam were born in 1969. Grandpa died two weeks later from nothing. They were both about eighty-five years old. They had a good, simple life and raised two good boys who gave them five grandchildren. I have often wished that they could come back, even for a day, to see the world now and to see their great- and great-great-grandchildren. They would need to see Phoenix, Los Angeles, Yorktown, and all the traffic. They would be surprised that Yorktown and Page Center were not the hub of the world, and that the whole world was not Lutheran. They would think that we were being lazy for getting all of our food from the grocery store and would not believe the fields of produce in California and Arizona and South America. I doubt they had ever seen a divided highway. The advances in farming and farm machinery would blow them away. Grandpa would think that there was no future in terraces and no-till farming. It would be a very busy day.

Grandpa was a "no nonsense, take no prisoners, just deal with it" kind of guy. That may have just reflected the pioneer attitude of his early years. Grandma would say "Ach, Charlie," in trying to counter some of his directness and empty threats. They drove a Ford coupe, which would be recognized now as a very desirable car. He used a Ford tractor for his farming in later years.

Grandpa would have farmed entirely with horses in his active years. I can remember the first tractor on the place. It had lug wheels and no rubber, like some of the Amish still use. So, all of Grandpa's years of farming, and the first few years of Dad's, had to be done with horses. Learning to use mechanical power had to have been at least as difficult as learning computers in our generation. My dad's generation had to go from animal power, which had been used almost since time began, to the new oil-powered tools. It had to have been especially difficult, since few had much formal education. Dad had no high school education. How did they read the manuals and understand the use and upkeep of these new tools?

Dad, his brother John, and Grandpa would assist each other with heavy work, such as threshing or haying. Uncle John bought one of the first balers, which required one person to sit on each side of the hay as it was being pooped toward the backdrop zone. These two would pass baling wire through the hay so that each of the square bales could have two wires tied about it. On one particular day, they had fought the machine all morning, trying to get it to work properly, and they must have been discouraged. I'm sure they decided that harvesting hay the old way was better, as they would have had the job done already.

While walking to Uncle John and Aunt Olga's house for the usual large dinner, Dad and his hired help, Roy Palmer, who was quite a mechanic, dropped back. Dad asked Roy if he thought that he could fix the baler, and Roy said he could. Dad bought that baler from Uncle John over the noon meal for the sum of one hundred dollars. That made for some good stories and could have been a source of friction. I don't believe it made much difference who owned the baler. It still baled for all of them. I never did understand how all of this trading of labor worked, but it did. We helped Uncle John, Ivan Otte, and Lee Wagoner, and they helped us. I believe the secret was that no one kept any track. It worked much like a commune.

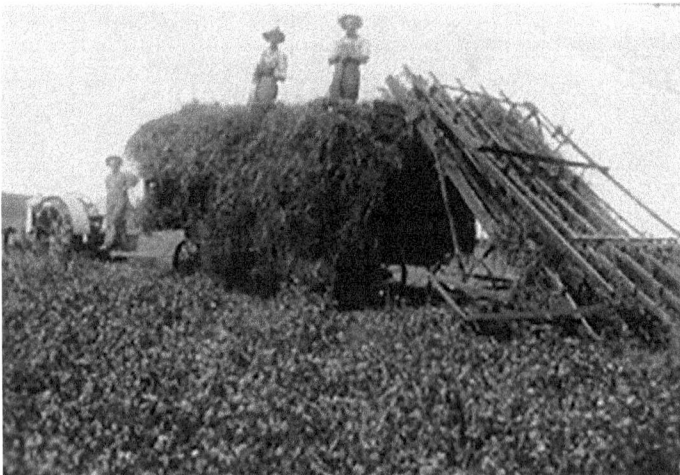

Making hay at the Otte farm. My dad, his brother John, and Grandpa Charlie at tractor. Note the hay loading contraption which brought the hay windrow up onto the hayrack thus avoiding having to pitch the hay up. They must have thought this was as good as it could get. Note the steel wheels with lugs on the tractor. It couldn't have been a smooth ride on the

road. The hay would've been taken to the haymow in a barn
or a haystack outdoors. There was no baling at this time.

The Ottes loved surprises and celebrations. They'd have a surprise celebration for the grandparents from about the twenty-fifth anniversary on, each time thinking that it would be the last—such celebrations were a Midwest custom. The family and friends would meet at a corner near the grandparents' place and, at the appointed time, would all drive as a parade to the home, honking and making as much noise as possible. That surprise would be considered very rude now, but it was the custom then.

Grandpa was never really sick or disabled, but he gradually spent more time on the "fainting couch" in their living room, and Grandma waited on him. I really haven't said much about Grandma, but she was always there in the background, letting Grandpa have the spotlight— as was the predominant custom then. Oh, for the good old days.

The family water system on our farm was an ingenious one created by our great grandfather Otte in the early 1900s. The main well for the farm was at the top of a gentle ridge, which ran about 150 yards west of the house. The slope from the house to the well was gentle, rising possibly ten to twenty feet in that distance. The well location, being elevated and away from the rest of the farm buildings, assured good clean water from the underground river which Grandpa said ran there. Indeed, I do remember neighbors coming to get water from that well in especially dry years. No pumps were available at that time, so it was necessary for pressure to be provided by gravity feed.

The elevation was not enough to provide the feed, so Grandpa invented a system to overcome that. He purchased a railroad tank car, cut off one end, then set it upright near the windmill with the open end to the top. He then covered it with a wooden lid. The windmill was able to fill that tank so that when the tank was full, it provided great water pressure for the farm and a volume of probably thousands of gallons of water. One can only imagine what a feat it must have been to raise that huge tank car and set it on end in cement with only the help of horses and a few neighbors. One can also imagine the party that must have been held at the Otte home that night. The people of that time were often pictured as stoic and deprived of fun, as in Grant Woods's *American Gothic* painting, but they knew how to party and used any excuse to do so. Where Grandpa got that tank car and why they were even available at that time, I'll never understand.

Windmills were quite common, but this one was a ways from the house. It was desirable to keep the tank nearly full so as to provide the best water pressure. For this to be accomplished, the windmill needed to be turned on (or in gear) or off as dictated by available winds and the needs for water. For convenience, then, a large-gauge wire was run from the windmill on/off handle to terminate at a windup mechanism held by several posts near the house. That was much better than walking the one-hundred-yard distance to the windmill each time it would need to be put in gear. It then became everyone's job to start or stop the pumping, depending upon needs and wind. We could tell that the tank was full only when it would run over. The youngest were not allowed to do this job, however, due to some "kick" in that winch mechanism. The windmill would also need to be shut off during high winds to avoid damage.

Here the story deteriorates. A hog house and feeding lot was placed around that tank sometime later, within ten feet of the windmill. I am convinced that some of that surface drainage found its way into the well water. The wooden cover on that tall tank also deteriorated through the years. The many birds in the area chose to sit on the edge around the top of that open tank. In later years it was decided to clean out the tank and replace the lid. I remember Dad's amazement at the two feet of sludge in the bottom of the tank. He surmised that this must have been from years and years of bird droppings. One can also imagine that the contents of the tank would have been stirred up each time the tank was filled. One also wonders what the original contents of that tank might have been and that some of the bottom contents would have been flakings from the inside of that container. The water always appeared clear and odorless and none of us became ill from the water, as far as we know. My sisters and I have often wondered now if some of that "stomach flu" that everyone would get at that time was from water or poor food preservation.

Still later, that system was changed so that the water was pumped directly from the well by an electric pump with a small reservoir. The windmill and tank car are no longer in use but remain in place today. The system was well ahead of its time.

My grandparents Mueller (my mother's parents) were William and Clara. I don't know as much about them, because Grandpa died while I was in grade school. Grandma Clara lived to be nearly one hundred years old. The only great grandparent on that side was Great Grandmother Goller, who was Clara's mother. I remember her only as being very old and always in a rocking chair at the Mueller place.

My mother's parents had five children: Martha (my mother), Paul, Carl, Wilma, and Eddie. The children were all born at California, Missouri, before the family moved to Clarinda, Iowa. Grandfather Mueller was a Missouri Synod Lutheran pastor and served approximately the last twenty years of his profession as pastor of Immanuel Lutheran Church, five miles northwest of Clarinda. Grandpa was well educated, having gone to school for as many years as a doctor, and he had some interesting hobbies. He collected coins, stamps, and local Indian artifacts, mostly arrowheads. He displayed the coins and some of the arrowheads in glass cases in their home. He loved to hunt duck and goose at Forney's Lake and took yearly vacations to Spirit Lake to fish. I still remember staying in the cabins at Spirit Lake. Grandfather was a terrible driver and would always rev his car to the maximum as soon as the starter turned it over. I don't remember Grandmother ever driving.

Grandfather Mueller was a strict "by the book" Lutheran minister. Communion was, thankfully, only once per month, but each communicant had to be counseled by him in his study the Saturday night before. His sermons were sometimes an hour long and were written out word for word. Some of his earlier sermons were given in German, and he was a pastor for the German prisoners of war in Clarinda during World War II.

The Mueller family Christmas gathering was at the parsonage during one of my preschool years. I was very excited about Santa Clause coming, whereupon Grandfather informed me that it would not be Santa, but the Holy Ghost. I surely did not want to see that guy, and the fact that I still independently remember the event testifies to its impact on my life. Grandmother Mueller took me aside later and assured me that it would be Santa coming, but we had been trained to respect Grandpa—so he was the one to believe. I don't remember if Santa ever did come that day. A child now would expect at least a support group or government grant for similar trauma.

Grandma served good meals for the Mueller gatherings, but Grandpa's table prayers were long. He would finish one prayer and then go right off into another. Being a good Lutheran, I knew them all by heart, so I knew what we were in for when he would start a new one. I have tried that same tack with our current grandchildren lately as a joke, but they won't stand for the long prayers like we did.

Grandfather Mueller retired from the ministry in the early 1940s and they moved to Yorktown, Iowa. He served as mayor of the town for some time and had a badge and small silver 32-caliber revolver as part of the office. They had a nice two-story house and several acres on the northwest edge of town. One Halloween, some of the town youngsters took Grandpa's goats and tied them to the flagpole in the center of town as a prank. I enjoyed visiting the Yorktown house because of the guns, artifacts, and Indian bow and arrow that Grandpa had. The rooms in the house were very small.

Grandpa died about five years after retiring to Yorktown. I was about twelve when he died. His body and casket sat in that small living room along the west wall. I always thought he died of heart failure, but several of his children have told me that he'd had strokes. After the first one, Dr. Bossingham told them that there would be two more and then that would be it. I surmise that he had atrial fibrillation or flutter and was in failure with that, and the strokes secondary to the dysrhythmia also hastened his death. They were probably not using anticoagulation for fibrillation or flutter at that time. I assume that my own atrial fibrillation was inherited from the Mueller side of the family.

After Grandfather's death, Grandmother Mueller (Clara) lived independently, then in apartments in Clarinda, and later in a nursing home. Grandmother had always been "just there" and took second place to Grandpa. The *Lutheran Witness* magazine was very important to her and may have been the only magazine she read. She had a funny butt wiggle when she walked, and I've wondered whether she had some congenital hip problem. She was a good lady and would hurt no one. I distinctly remember her crying hard while sitting at the foot of my mother's casket. Children should not die before their parents.

My Earliest Memories

I have been told that it is weird or impossible that I would remember such early events. I distinctly remember an early driving trip to St. Louis. I was sitting in the back seat of our car with Grandma Goller (Grandma Mueller's mother and my great grandma). I relayed this to my folks at a later age and they couldn't believe it because I was one year old when that trip was taken. I distinctly remember sitting in my wooden high chair with a one-inch wooden rim around the tray to hold the food in, and I was eating Pablum. I still remember the smell of that cereal and I don't like it. We recently found the spoon with the closed curved handle that I would have used.

I was convinced that I could lay eggs. I would squat and cackle— and the folks would slip eggs under me. I remember doing this act for company more than once. I could also run under the kitchen table without having to duck. This came in handy when running to avoid a spanking and was frustrating to the folks. My first remembrance of a lesson in not getting what I wanted was standing at the kitchen windowsill throwing a crying fit because Dad was driving to town and I wanted to go along. I don't know my age, but I was barely able to see out the window, even standing on tiptoes. I stood up in the pew at Immanuel once and loudly mocked or repeated back to Grandpa Mueller parts of his sermon. That was good for a spanking once we got home. The folks delayed the spanking sometimes so that I would have to think about it for a while. We had a family code word for needing to go to the bathroom while in public, and that word was "dodo" in our family. In my future wife Twyla's family, the words were "ba-ba" and "pee-pee."

I was sent to the ditch once to get a willow stick for my own spanking. The willow had lots of flexibility and seemed to develop some of its own energy on its way down to the butt. I'll bet I picked a small, weak switch. The willow trees seemed like magic to us because one can stick a branch into the ground and grow a new tree. I planted the twigs in a row across the stream to produce, eventually, willow-tree dams.

Soon after learning to walk, I started running away from home. That would cause an Amber Alert now, but no one came to get me, and I always returned home under my own power. I would frequently run to Ed and Mary Wagoner's home on the hill just east of our home. Mary would make me the best root beer, but the folks must have talked with her, because the root beers stopped. I also ran to visit Maxine and Ivan Otte's when they lived about a half mile northwest of our homeplace. The roads were not elevated at that time, so the road's bank extended upward from the road's surface. I found some wild strawberries on the bank on the east side of the road and sampled them. The berries were very small, but also the sweetest strawberries I have ever tasted. Maxine would occasionally feed me.

On another adventure, I was going down the long hill on the road just west of where Vera and Paul now live when a snake came out of the ditch on the north side of the road. It crossed in front of me, and its body was still coming out of the ditch on the north side while its head was already in the weeds on the south side. That was one long snake, even though the roads were not as wide then as later. I had a run-in with bumblebees on one of these trips but can't remember the details. The psychiatrists would call it suppression, but this might be the reason I'm so afraid of anything that stings now. I distinctly remember running away one day, intending to go to Uncle Otto's, about two miles to the southwest of home. I got to the bottom of their long driveway, lost my nerve, and ran back home. The folks asked where I had gone, and I got a whipping for lying. They didn't think I had been gone long enough to have made it that far.

The snows in those early years (1937–1939) seemed heavier, and maybe they were. At any rate, to a two- to five-year-old kid, the drifts seemed monstrous. I can still see how high the plowed roadside snow was, and it seemed three to four times my height—and maybe was. Those years produced heavy snows, as I understand. "Getting out" with the roads filled with snow or deep with mud, was frequent conversation. The roads were essentially trails, even though they were located on the mile lines, as surveyed much earlier. The road's surface was either flat with the terrain around or depressed. Snow and water would accumulate on the trail and make travel difficult. The farmers were pretty well saddled with maintaining their own roads. Much later, the roadways were elevated and "oiled" to make a firmer surface. That early oil was nothing like the current blacktop material, and I wonder whether it was just used oil from engines. Later, graveling was done, which is still the mainstay of all-weather roads in the area. The Q Road (running north off Hwy 2 toward Stanton) must have been elevated or hard-topped, because we knew that we could usually get as far as the mud road, the last half mile west to our home. Getting up Alfred's Hill (the first hill going west toward our home place) was always a worry. We would sometimes need to back up Ed Buch's hill to the east across the Q road and take a run through the stop sign for that first hill. It's not like there would have been much traffic at that stop sign in those years.

A two- to five-year-old kid would not have been much help to Dad on the farm, so we always had one or two hired men to help with the farm work. Dad had 200 acres to farm, and during World War II, he rented Uncle Carl's 160 acres directly west of the home place—in the quarter section on which Paul and Vera now live. This would have been considered a lot of land to farm at that time. Uncle Carl had bought that 160-acre farm as an investment when he went into the service, and Dad was to farm it. At one time there was a farm place on Uncle Carl's land where Vera and Paul live now. It had several barns and a house. We used the lower barn heavily to store hay, and it still stands today. The upper barn was near the road just east of the house and was quite an impressive structure. The bottom section was actually basement, built of local stones. On top of that foundation a tall barn was built, but we didn't use that barn much as it wasn't structurally sound above-ground. We stored the new combine in there, as it may have been the only building large enough to accommodate the machine. A large storm blew in one day, and Ivan Otte had the presence of mind—and the nerve—to drive the combine out just before the barn collapsed into a large heap of wood. That shiny red combine would have been in the basement among all that wood and it would have not been a "good thing." I believe the house on that farmstead had burned long before, so Dad chose that site to build a new house for the married hired help to occupy. I'm not sure why he placed the house on rented land, unless he thought that he would buy the 160 acres someday. Dad was unable to buy the farm when Uncle Carl sold it to Gene Otte, but some arrangement was made for Dad to buy the 5.08 acres that contained the house and some of the buildings. I distinctly remember the basement for that house being dug or cleaned out with a hand scraper—pulled, I believe, by a horse. I'm not sure whether the old burned-out foundation was used.

At times, Dad rented other farms around also. One was known as the Phillips place, in the section southeast of the famous Alfred's Corner. It had a farmstead then about an eighth of a mile back into the section, and some of the hired men lived there. It was necessary to cross a creek about fifteen feet deep in order to proceed up the long lane. The plank bridge across that creek was just that—planks—only with no side rails. It was only a single lane wide, and we always got a little rush when crossing the bridge, but we never ran off into the creek. At times horrendous floods would flow over the bridge on the creek, but I don't remember the bridge ever being taken out. The waterway is still there but has not flooded in later years—probably because of changes in farming practices and terraces. I specifically remember Chuck Moody (one of our hired men) picking a hundred bushels of corn by hand by noon, which was touted as some kind of record for hand-picking speed. Chuck had been a professional boxer and taught me some moves, but I thought he hit too hard. The second hired man at that time, Luther, lived on the Phillips place while the house and buildings were still there. One day, Luther's wife was sick, as well as one of his milk cows. Both the doctor and veterinarian were scheduled to visit, but Luther didn't know either of them by sight. When he arrived home at noon, he met the vet coming out of the house. The man carried a check, having just been paid by the wife. Luther naturally assumed that this was the human doctor, not the veterinarian who had just seen his wife. "How is she doing?" he asked. The vet answered, "Not so well. I think we will have to shoot her." This is a true happening, and Dad got lots of mileage out of this story. Dad did really enjoy the funny happenings in life that were mostly true. I'm not saying that Dad didn't embellish, but usually he didn't have to.

Our house had four bedrooms, and those were occupied, at times, by some of the hired help. The hired men thus became part of the family. There were times when two of the hired help at a time would live with us in our home, and they became a good part of my upbringing.

Many of the hired men later ended up being stable pillars of the community. Some of the names I remember are Charlie Schilb, Lawrence Reins, Clemon Wagoner, Paul Herzberg, and Bill Kirchner. Others came and went, including Luther, Chuck Moody, and Frank Svoboda. I distinctly remember when we picked up Frank Svoboda in Shenandoah. Dad knew nothing about his background and didn't ask. As a joke, Dad pulled into an especially dilapidated farmstead while taking Frank home, saying, "Here we are." Frank had a very solemn look on his face, as the selected farm was a run-down wreck, even at that time. He must have been relieved when we pulled up to the home place, one-and-a-half miles away, a beautiful, progressive homestead in comparison. Frank was a good worker, but did like to spend his weekends in Clarinda, probably at the bar, the Inda Clar, which is still going strong today. He eventually bought a Chevrolet coupe which must have been a girl magnet. I remember seeing that car, and it was pretty spectacular for the time. Dad loaned Frank two hundred dollars to buy the car. The next weekend, Frank didn't come home, and we have not heard from him or his two hundred dollars since. I have asked multiple Svobodas about it over the years, and none of them knew of a Frank. It seems that many Svobodas have been waitresses.

Ivan and Maxine Otte, who lived one-and-a-half miles west of us, had a different experience with hired help. They hired Bill, whom they knew nothing about, and he worked and stayed with them for the rest of his life. They often wondered what his real history was. Bill was a hard worker who spoke broken English, and I believe he was Czechoslovakian. He remained loyal to Ivan and Maxine and lived with them past Ivan's death and to his own. He faithfully attended our church and was buried in Immanuel cemetery, but he always maintained that he was Catholic. Bill said he was a sailor and, indeed, he could climb a rope easily and quickly using only his arms. He told us that his ship was on the ocean when the Titanic sank, and that they had heard the distress calls but were too far away to help. He was always a mystery, and I would like to know his true history. Bill could outwork any of the rest of us, and he seemed to be quite street smart but never got into any trouble. We sat and ate mulberries off the trees near the lower barn, just north of Paul and Vera's, as well as the world's best apricots from a tree at the old Bruce Wagoner place just south of their house. We would usually have some free time between loads of hay coming in to be put away in the haymow. Bill's idea of "pulling a calf" was to tie the presenting part of the calf to a tree and then scare the cow. Ivan and Dad didn't really approve of this method.

I would have been about four years old when my new sister, Irma, was brought home from the hospital. I distinctly remember Mother holding the new baby and that we were driving down Ed Buch's hill. We usually didn't take that road, but Dad must have thought it safer that day with the new baby—or perhaps we needed a "run" for Alfred's hill because of mud or, more likely, ice on that January day. It is strange that I don't remember much about Vera or Ruth as babies. I would have been in grade school by then and must have had other things to think about.

During World War II my toys were mostly guns and clothespin airplanes. I had a small machine-gun toy with a wooden ratchet that made a rat-tat-tat noise when the handle was turned. The other gun was a black plaster-of-paris pistol that looked like the ones used by Dick Tracy. I wish I still had them now. One of the hired men (Charlie Schilb, I believe) opened a door and crushed my Dick Tracy pistol. The folks said I should not ask him to replace the gun. Still worried that he would replace the gun with another type, I asked him one day, when the folks were not within hearing range, that if he were to replace the gun, to get exactly the same kind. The poor guy probably felt the pressure then, so he did get me a bigger pistol, which I never did like as well—and I probably let it be known.

Two of the old-fashioned clothespins made a good fighter plane, and three made a bomber. I had "airfields" of those planes hidden all over the house, and Mother was still finding those toys long after I was gone from home. I ran all about the farm buildings shooting my toy machine gun into the air when we heard the war was over.

Scrap metal was worth four cents per pound during the war, and I delighted in finding iron and adding to the scrap pile. I don't know what the arrangement was, but I'll bet I got paid in some way for what I contributed. It was a good feeling, knowing that more tanks and planes could be made out of my findings. Large "flocks" of B–29s flew over during the war, probably from Offutt air base, and I can still hear the loudness of the first jet.

I had a few toy trucks and cars about six-to-eight-inches long. A favorite pastime was playing in the dirt under an elm tree, grading roads and oiling them as was done to the real roads. Dad let me dip oil out of the barrel of used oil for this purpose. One of my toy cars stayed in the house. It had a spring mechanism that was, apparently, wound by pushing down on the back of the car. It would then run on its own for about twenty feet. Kids now would be amazed that I would have been amazed at that car. I recently bought a remote-control car for one of the grandchildren. It was from a kiosk at the Mall of America, and the salesman had it running all over the mall. I thought it would be something special for Ralph and something he'd never seen. Soon after that, I visited a toy store and found that one couldn't buy a car that was *not* remote-controlled. The kids would say "That's okay, Grandpa."

Food and gas stamps were all part of WWII, but I don't remember going without much. Bananas and flour were hard to get. Dad was happy to sell a load of corn on the black market for two dollars per bushel. It's amazing (and sad) that corn is still worth about that same amount now, sixty-five years later.

We had huge American Elm trees around the house. The largest was in the yard south of the house near the road. A strong, horizontal branch extended out south about twenty feet up the tree, and held a swing made with one-inch rope. This provided hours of entertainment and gave one heck of a swing. Dutch Elm disease felled all of these great trees some years later. Nothing is forever.

I don't know where it came from, but I had a peddle car that I loved. One could sit in it, but unfortunately, something was broken on the mechanism so it would not peddle. If Dad had known how much I wanted that car to go, I'm sure he would have fixed it. It was an orange color, and one day I decided to paint it white. It must have seemed like too big a job for a five-year-old, as all our pictures of the car show only one brush swipe of white paint across the grill.

Dad had quite a business going at one time. Folks would bring their horses or mules over to be bred by our Jack, which I guess was just one huge donkey. He had a special chute in which this activity would occur, and then people would take their animals back home. I don't know what I thought went on but am sure I didn't understand it. I remember asking Dad what the bull was for, and he said that the bull helped with the calves being born. I must have assumed that the bull was some kind of midwife.

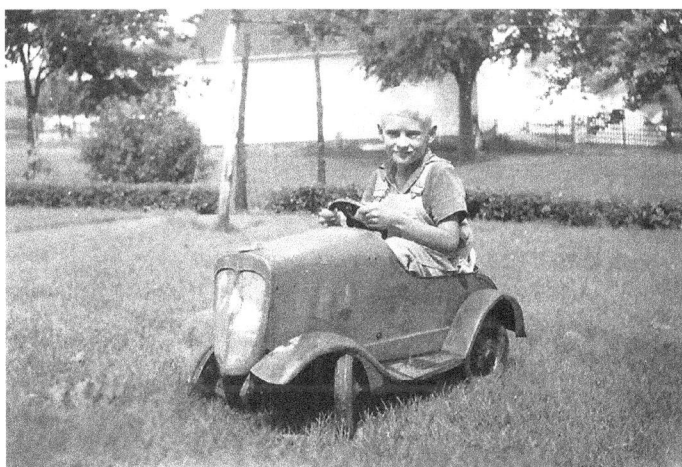

This is a peddle car I wanted badly to work. I don't know where we got it, but it was probably given to us. If Dad had known how much I wanted the car to work, I'm sure he would

Dad made homemade beer and wine. We even had our own bottle capper. One night, we were all sitting out in the yard (the folks and the two hired men and myself) when we heard the beer bottles breaking from too much of something, probably sugar, in the beer. In order to save the homemade brew, they opened all the bottles and emptied them into a large crock so it could be dipped out into glasses and consumed. There were several happy hired men that night, and I think I even got a few sips. Dad kept the beer and wine in our cave, which was deep and cool—probably around a constant sixty degrees.

Before rural electricity, we had an upright icebox at the west end of that long, screened porch and just outside the side entrance to the kitchen. We would buy several fifty-pound ice blocks on Saturday night that would keep food cool in the icebox for at least part of that week. The ice blocks, I am told, would be cut from the river or lake in the winter and somehow preserved in that large cooler building in Clarinda across from the Opitz Ford Motor Company.

A small community-owned butcher house with a large butcher block was located just off the north–south road east of Vera and Paul's place. It was owned cooperatively by twenty-two families. A calf would be butchered there early every Sunday morning, and families would pick up their share of fresh meat. I'm sure most of the meat would then be kept in some type of icebox at their homes, to be consumed during the early part of each week. Once the REA (rural electricity) came to the farms, people got refrigeration and there was no need for the weekly slaughter. The little building then sat empty for many years until it was finally torn down, probably about the time Gene Otte bought that farm. I hope the butcher block was saved somewhere, as it would be a great antique now.

Mother prepared all steak the same way and called it minute steak or round steak. We had never heard of T-bone steak, so much of that fried steak must have been choice cuts of very fresh meat. It would be fried, and gravy made, which was applied to potatoes or broken-up slices of bread. I liked to cut the meat into small pieces and mix it in with the gravy and bread. Twyla tried to reproduce that meal for years after we were married. We bought round steak and minute steak, but it just wasn't the same. One of my sisters told us that we needed to fry T-bones, and sure enough, that was it. There was no barbecue early on, so everything was fried or cooked, even the best cuts. I'm happy with Twyla's steaks now that we are frying our T-bones.

We had a phone as far back as I can remember, but they were a large piece of furniture hung on the wall and powered by two big, oblong, cylindrical batteries. The phone lines all ran to Yorktown where an operator would dispatch the calls twenty-four hours per day. We would be mindful not to place calls too late at night, as one lady did all of this from her home; and besides, the ring would be heard by all who were on that line. We were on a party line of about eight families and could call anyone on that line without going through the switchboard. Each party would have a distinctive ring made up of very subjective short and long rings produced by turning the handle either a long time or short time. We were a long and a short, but realistically everyone listened to all the calls on their own party line anyway. I believe that these were the earliest phones and would certainly have been a big advancement over no phone at all.

Farmers did general farming in those early years, from 1936 to 1942. We raised corn, oats, milo, several grasses, and several kinds of hay. We all had cattle, hogs, and chickens. Some of the roosters could be quite mean, and I was frightened of them. I had a new set of white overshoes of which I was very proud. The first day, I walked in them in mud near the chicken house. A large rooster came at me and I jumped right out of those boots and ran to the house. Mother held me up to the north window of the kitchen, and I could see those boots standing upright there in the mud. I must have thought the rooster would eat my new boots.

Dad got a hand infection sometime in the early war years and was in the Clarinda hospital with his hand elevated and hot-packed. He was treated with a sulfa drug, which was very new then. He took a number of the pills every three hours and recovered well. I believe this was just before penicillin.

Visiting was done by simply getting in the car and going to surprise someone. Maybe this was a holdover from having no phones. If one family was not home or didn't answer, we would go to another place to visit. On one very cold night we drove to Uncle Otto's to visit. I had the croup, so mother told me to keep my mouth shut on the way to the house. Dad then said to keep it shut inside the house too. I had to have been very young, but that remark has stayed with me. We were to be seen and not heard.

Before balers, hay would be put into the barn loose, or stacked outdoors. The hay would be stomped down as much as possible by the people, either in the barn or on the stack. When finished, the stack would be a pretty shape, compact and able to shed water. The work was very labor-intensive, so the German prisoners of war were a godsend during the war years. On hay or threshing days, Dad would go to the prison camp and bring home up to four prisoners for a day's work on the farm. The prisoners worked hard and loved coming, as they got good German food and could talk German with the farmers. They even got some beer. No guards were sent with the prisoners and none ever escaped. These men were just not much into the war. They worked with any tools they needed, including pitchforks and machetes, but I don't remember having any fear of them. Some of the prisoners made us some authentic German items. I remember especially one of those chicken paddles that when put into motion, looked like chickens feeding off the ground. They also made some beautiful colored rings out of plastic—play toys that were works of art. I wish we still had these. Mom loved feeding the German prisoners, as they were so appreciative. The Japanese prisoners were always sent to work with guards, and we never had any of the Japanese to help us.

Many children go through a biting stage. I remember that we visited Lawrence Reins's family when they lived in the starter house east of the church. I must have been about five or six years old and had a disagreement with Gerhardt such that I bit him hard enough to leave tooth marks. When that bite mark got shown to the adults, my folks bit me equally hard right there on the spot. I believe that cured any urge I might have had to bite anyone in the future.

Lee and Marion Wagoner's wedding was celebrated after church at the Ed Wagoner homeplace—the first place east of ours. I was preschool age at that time and rather scrawny. Children were allowed much more freedom in those days, and at gatherings like this, would be allowed to play all over the farm—including climbing anything and visiting any of the farm buildings. Two older boys were acting like bullies and giving me a bad time that night. I complained to the adults, including Lee, the groom (as if he would have time) and got no help. I don't know why I didn't just stay at the house with the adults. The next time these two boys caught me, I was in the east end ground floor of the corn crib. They came into the building from the west and I had no way out. They were threatening to beat me up. A full-sized axe leaned against the wall near me. It would have weighed about a quarter of my weight, but I lifted it and rushed the boys. They retreated quickly, and I had no more trouble with them that night—or ever.

The folks were in a group that met each Fourth of July. Besides the folks, the group included the families of Paul Mueller, Lawrence Reins, Ivan Otte, Melvin Royer, Norman Carlson, and sometimes other invitees. Food, liquor, and fireworks were plentiful. We were allowed to do some of the fireworks when we were quite young, and I don't know why we didn't have more injuries or fires. We *held* the Roman candles as they were shot off and blew up everything we could with those increasingly powerful, large red firecrackers (M–80s or something similar). One time in later years at our place, there was more drinking than usual, and I was embarrassed for my dad. I took Dad's Seagram's Seven bottle and hid it on the top shelf of my closet where it stayed for years. I took the bottle with me later to school in Des Moines where it provided sips for me for a long time.

Grade School Years

Both Twyla and I attended Immanuel Lutheran Grade School for the entire nine years, primary through eighth grade. The school was a solid, rectangular red brick building which sat at the top of the hill in the empty lot south of the present church. There was a home for the principal, who also taught, between the present church and the school. The school building sat on several acres, with a wide expanse of grass and trees spread across the grounds. Two ball diamonds were separated by a tall fence-like backstop. The smaller ball field, used by the "little room" students, primary through fourth grade, was to the west. The "big room" diamond, used by grades five through eight, lay to the east. The principal, Mr. Schamber, taught these older grades. A good metal swing set and a wooden teeter-totter provided good entertainment. A pair of two-holer outdoor privies—one for boys and one for girls—sat back a ways. The boy's toilet also had a U-shaped fence attached to the east side which held a tin trough tilted toward the privy and which drained into the hole beneath the toilet. This was for urination only. A favorite sport was to wait until the boys would have a stream going and then give them a good shove which would cause an embarrassing wet spot on the jeans for the rest of the day. My sisters remember toilet paper being rationed, two sheets for each trip to the toilet.

A small wooden shed with a low A-frame roof just north of the school building provided many hours of time for the game called Anti-over. The two teams would be on opposite sides of the roof and one would throw a volleyball over so that it had to bounce off the roof on the other side. If the ball was caught, the team could come around and try to capture as many of the other team as possible by hitting them with the ball. If the ball was not caught, the ball needed to be returned over the roof so that the first team would have their chance to catch it and do the same. The teams changed sides each time the ball was caught. Members of the team being chased would be safe once they reached the opposite side of the building. There was a large half-circle drive-through on the west of the school where parents could park. There were no marked parking spots and always plenty of room. No one had to park on the road. I didn't realize that this was such a big deal until recently when I experienced the congestion at the Scottsdale schools.

Twin metal shoe scrapers were located at the front entrance to the school building. These were made of two four-foot-long, quarter-inch-thick strips of iron embedded in cement, laid longitudinally and protruding about four inches above the cement. A very strong hand grip made of one-and-a-half-inch pipe extended upward for about three feet at each end of the scraper, connected by the same pipe. We spent hours rotating on that crossbar and I don't know why someone didn't split their head by falling on that scraper.

Upon entering the front (west) side of the building, one came into a landing about ten feet square. Straight ahead was a wide set of about nine steps leading to the upper level and then a smaller landing with three exits. Straight ahead was the hall-type coat room with clothing hooks along both walls and a long wooden hall tree down its center. This imposing piece of furniture was accessible from both sides for hanging coats and boots and had a full-length eye-level shelf for lunch pails. To the right was the "big room" for grades five through eight. To the left was the "little room" for primary through fourth grade.

Back now to the aforementioned landing inside the entrance. Off to the left of that area, a long set of perhaps twenty steps led to the basement. These steps were narrow and quite steep, as it was a long way down. The actual basement room was off to the right of the landing, with a curtain entrance. The front of each step was either metal-capped or very slick wood. I discovered that, with my slick leather shoes, I could "ski" down the fronts of the steps, touching only the very front edge of each step, with my right hand on the handrail for stability. I could be down into the basement within several seconds with this technique. God help anyone who would come through that curtain onto the landing during my descent. The building had a full garden-level basement with a nice wooden floor and basketball hoop at the north and south ends, and perhaps a twenty-five-foot-high ceiling. There was also a furnace room, but no air conditioning. The entire south end of that basement was a stage—complete with side dressing rooms and a very nice curtain which would open and close for stage action. The basement was about thirty-by-sixty feet in size and had high windows to the outside.

That school basement provided a nice place to play during the many bad outdoor days of the school year. A volleyball net would sometimes go up in the middle of the room. I have many good memories of these activities. I don't know firsthand, but rumor was that unapproved boy–girl activities took place in the furnace room and behind the stage walls and curtain. Twyla says she was careful never to be caught behind the stage. Mr. Schamber, the big-room teacher, would go to his home at noon, leaving the fifty students to be supervised by the small-room teacher—but I don't remember much supervision.

The school basement served as a multipurpose room. The school Halloween activities were always fun. Straw would be brought in for tunnels, and there were always some scary areas. Apple-bobbing was an annual attraction. The Walther League would present an annual play, and the basement could seat several hundred people for the performance. Early on, travel movies would be shown on the 16-mm school projector, a big event for the community. The school children would present an annual end-of-school-year program in the basement on the stage. These programs would consist of skits, patriotic singing, and much student talent.

Besides the official program, an annual softball game would be held on the last day of the school year between Immanuel and St. Paul's school in Yorktown. The ball games were a political thing, and our pitcher pretty well determined who would be on the team of nine. No effort was made to allow all to take a turn at play, as those end-of-school-year games were quite serious. Only the best players were chosen, and they played all nine innings. I had good moments but was not a good enough player to make any of the big games. They even loaned me to the Yorktown team one year when that team did not have nine players. The competition on the Immanuel team was stiff, as we had some very good athletes, such as Donald and Eugene Otte, Harry Bar, Dean Sunderman, Ermal Herzberg, Willard Herzberg, and Cecil and Paul Sunderman.

Basketball games with Yorktown were intermittent during the winters. Raymond Buch was our coach and I must have been allowed to play at least once. I remember getting confused and making a basket for the opposing team once. The coach wrote a summary of each game, then posted it on the bulletin board at school the next day. He mentioned that goof in his report and stated that Carl should have been pulled from play immediately. That comment, posted on the board at school, hurt me deeply.

The school board was tasked with setting up a large refreshment stand for this Sunday event at the end of the school year. The stand sold everything a kid would like, at a good price. All students received a number of five-cent tickets from the school to be used at that stand. It was truly a magical day for us, and we really looked forward to the event. We all felt much relief at being done with the stress of the program, knowing that we passed that grade in school. I vividly remember not knowing whether I had passed fifth grade arithmetic until the day of the program.

Immanuel Lutheran School consistently had about fifty students, and it was a relief for everyone when the weather was warm enough that we could play outdoors. The most common activity centered around the two softball fields. The games of "tag" and "chain" were also popular activities.

The church had a parsonage for the minister and a nice house for the school principal, both located between the school and church. A long barn divided the two homes and housed the horses many of the students rode to school. My early grade school years marked the end of that era, as car travel would soon take over as the preferred mode of travel.

Sometime during that car-travel time, my mother was returning home from delivering the oldest of us three to Immanuel School when Ruth fell out of the moving car. She was only three years old. We had Chrysler or Desoto cars then, with the "suicide doors" for the rear seats. That meant that the hinges were on the back of the doors so that they swung open from the front. Thus, if the door was open even a little, the wind of the car's forward motion would pull the door open quite strongly. Ruth was riding in the back seat on the way home, unrestrained, which was common for that time period. She opened the door. Mother heard the wind, looked back, and saw the open door with Ruth hanging on to the inside door handle. They were driving on the Q road which was hard surfaced by then, and Mother had the presence of mind to slow and pull over to the right, where Ruth fell into the ditch. She sustained some pretty bad facial abrasions from the weeds, but no serious injuries—unless they haven't shown up yet. Mother took Ruth to the Clarinda Hospital (at a little higher speed, I'm sure). A local doctor, whom the folks did not care for, was at the hospital. He cleaned her up and took credit for saving her life. I don't believe Ruth needed any stitches, and she has no scars from this, that I know of. I don't remember whether she was admitted.

Can you imagine parents now allowing their grade-school-age kids to ride a horse for up to five miles to school? I remember very well housing my pony in that barn during my second- to fourth-grade years. We lived three-and-a-half miles from school, but many of those who lived closer just walked. It was sport for some of the walkers to throw dirt clods and rocks at my pony to scare him. This was very frightening to me. I would try to get on the road home before the walkers or take a longer way home. I remember even now who the students were who would scare my horse in that way. One of my ponies was small, black, and quite nervous. Cars would spook him, so sometimes I would walk him along the fences to be as far as possible from the road. I fell off one time after one of his lunges, and my foot went forward through the stirrup as I fell. I was dragged for a ways under the pony, and I remember the animal stepping on my face. No one came to save me, but the horse eventually did stop. I was able to free myself and ride the rest of the way home. I don't know if anyone believed my story or understood how dangerous the situation had been.

Grandfather Mueller (Mother's dad) was minister of Immanuel Lutheran Church for about twenty years, which ended during my early grade-school years. I stayed at the parsonage with the grandparents during my primary-school year (about age five or six) and the folks would take me home for the weekends. The parsonage was a large square house with four bedrooms upstairs. I slept in one of the south bedrooms. There was no heat upstairs, except that which came up through the floor grates from downstairs. Grandmother would heat old irons and wrap them and place them in bed with me at my feet. Those were a welcome sign of love and caring. Grandfather was a different story, and I must have been frightened of him. He was a strict, stubborn German who would have thought it a weakness to show any love. He had a large garden and a barn with about four milk cows, so he was a hard worker in addition to his duties as minister. He was, however, a terrible driver. He would race the engine of his Plymouth at its maximum RPM as part of his starting routine. That car had to have suffered due to all that revving before oil got to the pistons.

Grandpa crossed the center line once, sideswiping Dad in our old black Desoto on Hwy 2 near Alvie Sunderman's place. Dad told about the investigating officer asking the usual questions. When he got to "Do you know each other?" Dad said, "Yes, he is my father-in-law." The officer put his pad away and said, "You two just settle this."

The minister would have been the most educated person in the community by far, so he engendered much respect and admiration. To attend a social event with the minister or to have him over for a meal was an absolute highlight to be savored for a long time.

I was sent to Center School, a one room public school about a mile-and-a-half from home on Snake Creek, for my first-grade year. I don't know why I went there instead of Immanuel—perhaps because it was closer. A large buckskin horse was my usual mode of transportation. I don't remember a horse barn there, so I must have tied the horse to a fence or tree for the school day. The dinner pail would usually hold chocolate milk, and the ride would actually churn butter in that thermos. We had only whole milk then, so it is easy to see how butter could appear in that bottle. I remember being so very proud that I had actually made something with my ride, but it probably meant that I was just not a very smooth rider. I got so mad at Leonard Sump once for naming his horse the same as mine that I hit him. Both of our horses were huge animals. We were visiting one day at the bottom of the Sump lane when the two horses decided to race. They took off at full speed, with us on their backs, until they reached Alfred Sump corner, nearly a half mile down the road. Neither of us fell off, but it would not have been good if we had.

The names of my horses escape me, probably because I had so many, though only one at a time. It seemed that my horse was always dying. Dad said that it was because the horses were not of good quality. He said he usually bought a saddle and they would throw a horse in with it. It could be that the older horses were used for the kids to ride, as they would be tamer and not likely to run so fast.

Center School was a typical one-room country school, with the potbelly stove near the back of the room. There had to be a large variance in temperature in that room. The kids with desks toward the back had to have been hot, while those in front were cold. I was usually at one of the front desks. Outdoor clothing and dinner buckets would be hung on hooks along the back wall. There were fewer than ten pupils in the entire school.

One day, we made fudge as a class project. It was placed in an open window to cool. Leonard and I snuck out the back and ate some of the candy off the plate from the outside. I'm sure we were punished, but I don't remember how. At another time, I had thrown a large number of snowballs into the girls' outhouse. This was reported to the teacher and I was sent out, during class time, to clean out the girls' biffy. I thought that was great, as I never got to go in there any other time. Once I got in trouble for throwing a huge ice ball—not a snowball—from close range at one of the Claybaker boys. For this, I was locked in the woodshed. Fortunately, I found an axe inside, so I chopped my way out and went home. Mabel, Twyla's mother, loves to tell a story about one of the Sunday afternoon parties for Center School students and parents. She said they heard a hissing sound and found me letting air out of the car tires.

At one of these parent gatherings, a fruit jar was buried near a large post on the east fence. Everyone placed an object or note in the bottle, intended to be recovered in some later year. Dad wrote that he thought the war would be over. I don't know that the bottle has ever been recovered. The school's land has been sold and fencing changed. Given the size of that post, we would never have guessed that we could not find the burial site at a later time.

Center School was closed the next year, I believe, and that would explain why I went back to Immanuel for the second grade. I'm glad I was allowed to pass the first grade, as my antics must have been a rebellious stage for me. Some years later the Center School building was washed away by a flood on Snake Creek.

Immanuel provided my education from second through eighth grade, and I believe they did their job well. Many of the roads, which are hard-surfaced now, were non-elevated dirt roads—paths. At times Dad would take me to the intersection of the Q road and Kenneth Sunderman's road (near where Paul lives now) and from there I would ride the last mile to school with the Albert Herzberg kids in their buggy. That makes me think that the last mile to school must have been a dirt or mud road. Later, we traded transporting kids with Herbert Sumps by car. I don't remember ever walking all the way to school. Grandpa Mueller must have retired around the time of my second-grade year, and that ended the option of staying with them.

My favorite time in the little room, other than recess, was story time. This took place immediately after noon recess. The teacher would read a good book to the class in successive segments for about fifteen minutes each day. Valentine's Day in those years was a big deal. We would buy books of valentines which we would punch out. Then we'd carefully select which verse to give to whom. One of those years, I remember buying three special cards for about ten cents each for Martha, Marnice, and Wanda. I handed the cards to each on Valentine's Day and then ran away. I'm not sure why I chose them to get the real cards, except that maybe they were a little more "developed" than the rest of the girls in the room.

Wanda Otte was a delightful second cousin of mine. She was always a little bigger and louder than others and appeared to have more fun. Wanda sat directly in front of me in the second grade. Our desks had seats that folded up and left about a one-inch opening between the hinges. One day (for what reason, I don't know) I poked Wanda's behind rather hard through that crack in the back of the seat with my sharp compass point. Wanda, being her bashful, quiet self, immediately stood bolt upright and screamed that she had been hurt in her behind—by me. Florence, the teacher, had to respond, so she made me stay after school, which was probably a first for me. She spoke with me about it, and I was devastated. To make matters worse,

Florence later married my future wife's uncle, Otis, and we spent considerable time with Uncle Otis and Aunt Florence through the years. She was very gracious in saying that she did not remember the event. I don't believe the incident scarred Wanda too much. She became a strong business person in Clarinda with her recycling business and occasionally assisted her son, Jay, with his funeral business. Wanda has made delicious cakes for local events for years; in fact, she made our wedding cake in 1961.

The big room teacher for grades five through eight, Mr. Schamber, was a strict taskmaster and even stricter Lutheran. He ruled by fear but did the very best he could and was a good person. He was just not warm and fuzzy. His teachings apparently took well with me, and I spent most of my waking time worrying about not being good enough to go to heaven if I should die at that moment. We were told not to think about girls, so I quickly banished any thought or mind picture of a girl. I didn't really understand, I guess, what it was about girls that we were to avoid. If not for this fear, Twyla and I might have started dating in grade school. Sexual sins were given such high priority, and I had the feeling that those sins would place one on a slippery slide straight to hell. The moment of death was apparently a pivotal point in God's judgment of the person, and actually counted for everything.

Mr. Schamber was unquestionably a good person, although very compulsive. His entire life had been spent teaching, and I don't feel he could have had much fun. No one else seems to remember, but I recall him saying that sex, even in marriage, should be undertaken only to reproduce and not for pleasure. I don't remember him ever telling a joke. I told him once that I did not like that large dictionary in the back of the room because it said Carlsbad (New Mexico), which I took to be a play on my name. He seemed to enjoy that statement and repeated it often to people as a very clean joke.

Mr. Schamber did all the chores and upkeep at the school—at least what he could not get us to do. He was in charge of building maintenance and cleaning as well as teaching. Student help in these areas was, indeed, part of our education. He was a pretty good piano player and accompanied for school and church events. He also played the organ for church each Sunday. He had to play the organ for funerals too, so when they occurred, school was put on hold and the kids just sang for each funeral. We all fondly remember the musical programs at the end of the school year and the huge children's program each Christmas Eve, but we grew sick of attending funerals.

Two events stand out in my memory from the big room. One is watching the Emil Sunderman home burn from our south windows. The home was on a hill about one mile south of the school, so was easily observed by all of us as it burned to the ground. I didn't know at that time that I would marry their granddaughter. Twyla was eight years old and remembers that the students in the little room were allowed to come into the big room to watch out the south windows.

The second event was the day someone came to the door to get Cecil and Paul when their dad, Wilbert, was killed. I've always felt bad about saying "you lucky guys" as they left the room, not knowing at that time the reason for their summons.

Mr. Sunderman, Cecil and Paul's dad, had been killed in a field about a quarter mile north of the school in a tractor accident. He had been doing some work on a dam with his tractor and a manure scoop. The combination of a loaded elevated scoop and uneven ground caused the tractor to roll. An ambulance had gone by the school earlier with its siren wailing. That ambulance noise was a one-time event, but we didn't realize its significance until later in the day. That accident and the funeral had a profound effect on us at school because it affected some of our own so deeply. The bodies, at that time, were embalmed and kept in the home until the church funeral. Mr. Sunderman's casket was displayed in a small room just off the kitchen. He was buried in the Clarinda cemetery, possibly because their farm was so close to the Immanuel cemetery and actually overlooked it. I remember being stressed about how to address the subject with Cecil and Paul in the time after the death.

Confirmation classes were taught by the minister in our seventh- or eighth-grade year. These classes, taught by Pastor Kreutz, took place for an hour each morning in a tiny room just off the small room. The purpose was to instruct us in the Missouri Lutheran beliefs, with the end point being our affirmation or confirmation of such in front of the congregation on Confirmation Day.

We had practically memorized Luther's Catechism and would be expected to recite large parts of it on that day. We put ourselves through much stress as we worried about embarrassing ourselves in front of everyone we knew. The class would be seated on chairs in the front of the church and questioned for up to an hour. It was and is definitely a dress up and picture day and usually a contest over which family had the minister over for the large meal after church. The day is important enough to Lutherans that their obituaries usually give the day of confirmation as well as who presided over it.

Graduation from the eighth grade presented another stressful situation. Those in country schools had to take a county test administered by the county superintendent, to see if they were qualified to go to the high school in Clarinda. Some were worried enough about this test that the parents would transfer a child to Clarinda schools earlier in order to avoid the test. Twyla and Ardith took that test and tied for second in the county. I registered somewhere below them. It was one of the few tests that Twyla and I have had to compete in, except for driving tests.

During this grade school time, the folks bought a Doodlebug motor scooter for me at Gambles in Clarinda for $129. We visited with Uncle John later that day, and I was so excited about the scooter that I blurted out the purchase and the cost. The folks were so angry about that revelation that they threatened to take the scooter back—which they didn't. I spent hours of my childhood riding that machine, but never went too far from home with it. We could not keep the gasoline from leaking out the bottom of the tank, and the machine spent much time in Roy Palmer's shop as he tried to keep it running. It still provided many hours of fun—and I had something that no one else did. We have a considerable number of early home movies of this Doodlebug.

CHAPTER TWO

High School Years

All seven students from our Immanuel eighth grade went to high school. It was somewhat of a culture shock to have classes without the biblical slant—especially science classes. We had been taught not to dance or worship with those of other faiths. This admonishment set us up to fail socially. Some of the other strengths of our training, though, were good, and all Immanuel's students were well accepted. Some of us did quite well in sports, but others found it not their strong suit. Most of the boys from the country schools were expected to help with the farm work, and this made it difficult to stay after school for sports practice.

Ours was one of the last classes to have the ninth grade in the old junior high, located just north of the sports field. The building was later condemned and taken down. Grades ten, eleven, and twelve happened at the Clarinda High School—which has also been removed and the new library built in its place. The new high school and sports facilities are now west of Clarinda.

At first, my mode of transportation to the town schools was the yellow school bus. Later, I rode with Gene Otte, who had his own car. My folks paid Gene or his parents something like twenty-five cents per day for transporting me. Gene was a good friend, so I actually enjoyed that—and I hope Gene and Wanda did too. We once slid off a very slick Q Road into soft snow on the west side. The car was laid on its left side into a drift in the ditch and had no damage. There were no cell phones, so I assume someone must have come along and given us a ride. We would have known most everyone traveling the Q Road at that time.

The folks and I thought we owed Gene a good Christmas gift since he was so good to us. We gave him a hood ornament consisting of a bull's head with ivory-like horns about two inches long that would light up. I have always felt bad about that gift, as it was one of those things that he just about had to use. The gift had to be installed and hooked into the electrical system of the car. Gene never indicated that he didn't like the gift. It made his Chevrolet very distinctive, and no one else had one.

I had no car and the folks were not big on transporting me to social activities and games. I don't remember them ever going to see a sporting event or even attending the track meets in which I participated. Arnold Dammann had his own maroon jeep and he and Gene were very good at taking me to evening events. In the last year or two of high school, I was allowed to drive the family car or our old red pickup. I did much of my dating in that pickup. It was not much of a chick magnet.

Our mode of dress for grade school was overalls, complete with bib. We have the film from when Dad took home movies of all the students at Immanuel. I was the only one who knew the pictures would be taken that day, so I wore a *tie* with my bib overalls. The dress for high school and junior college would have been jeans. My jeans sustained an acid spill in junior college chemistry lab, but I continued to wear them to school, as I can see in old pictures. My waist size was 28–30 then and remained so for ten years until I left general practice in 1973 for the emergency department residency.

Junior high, ninth grade when I started, seemed so big and intimidating to us country folk. One pivotal event in the ninth grade started my political career in high school. Mrs. Clements, teacher of ninth-grade English, asked that each student write what they did during the last summer and read that essay to the class. I dutifully wrote about my summer activities on the farm in a most serious manner. I didn't intend for the writing to be funny, just factual. The writing was about farm work combined with time off for fishing at the ponds, hunting and trapping, butchering, milking, and catching mice.

I told about raising "Elsie the Dirty Pig," who was my hog. Dad provided the feed and space and I was allowed to keep any profits from her and her brood. She had several litters per year, all on her own, without any input from us. She would just go out somewhere and come home later with ten or eleven little pigs. This simplicity must have hit a funny bone with the town kids, as they would not quit laughing at my serious presentation. Because it was so well received, Mrs. Clements arranged for me to read my essay to all of her other English classes. I soon found myself the homeroom president.

Each homeroom was responsible for one program at assembly. I wrote a humorous school play that included both pupils and teachers, making use of some of the joke books that were part of Dad's magic materials. That went well, and I was soon class president—quite a feat for a simple country boy from Immanuel Lutheran School.

I went on to become vice president my sophomore year and class president junior year. I remember that well because the juniors plan the senior prom, and that was a lot of work. Being junior class president, I chaired the meeting for election of senior officers. For senior president, there was a tie between Merle Eberle and me. I wasn't sure how to handle that, so I, being the current president and the one running the election meeting, broke the tie by proclaiming Merle the winner. He was a real jock and deserving of the honor. He stayed in Clarinda after high school and ran the A's baseball program and has been a great asset to the town.

I was no good at sports. Basketball was a laughing matter, and at 140 pounds, I didn't even bother to think of football. I was okay at track, probably because of all the running I did to get our dumb milk cows from the furthest corner of the pasture. I was on our two-mile relay team that set the Iowa record for that race in 1955. The record stood only one year and was broken the next year, after I graduated—

by the same team—without me. There were four of us who could run near two-minute half miles in 1955. I never did get below two minutes, but I came close many times.

Speaking of milk cows, ours had to have been the dumbest ones on the planet. They would congregate as far from the barn as possible at milking time each night and would not answer any call. I threw a rock at one once and it hit the cow on the top of the head in the horn area. The cow dropped like a rock, and I was sure that I had killed it. It lay there for a while and finally did get up. I don't know if I ever told Dad about that.

We had no milking machines in the '50s, so we milked anywhere from one to four cows by hand. We would wash the teats off with water if they looked dirty and then set the bucket under the udder and milk manually. The bottom of the bucket always contained a little dirt, so we wouldn't pour out the very bottom of the milk. We would keep some for our own use and separate the cream out of the rest to sell in town on Saturday night. We had no pasteurization, and I don't know why we didn't get sick.

In those days we used DDT heavily for fly control. I remember an open can of DDT sitting on a shelf in the barn. We'd paint the DDT on the wall with a brush so we could watch the flies land on the wall and fall dead. We also painted the DDT on the side of the cow next to where we sat, so as to discourage flies sitting there while we milked. It was fun shooting the milk stream toward the cats, and they got pretty good at opening their mouths and catching the stream in midair. I have recently read that cow's milk is bad for cats. Maybe that is why they always had diarrhea.

Some of the cows wouldn't stand still to be milked, so we would apply "kickers" around their back legs in order to restrain the rear leg motion. Many times, the cow would step into the bucket, and then we'd have to discard that bucket of milk. One time I had a brand-new coat—which didn't happen often enough—of which I was very proud. My girlfriend at that time was Jan Braymen, and she was out to the farm to watch me milk the cows. I wore the coat that evening. Applying kickers requires one to bend under the cow's rear to affix the kicker on the left leg and then pass the chain ahead of the legs and attach the cup around the right leg. This requires that the operator spend some time behind and below the tail of the cow. The first cow happened to have severe juicy diarrhea just as I reached behind to apply the kickers. Liquid cow stool thus covered my hair and, worst of all, my new coat. The very worst part, though, was hearing Jan laugh uncontrollably. I was so embarrassed. But I wore that silly stained coat for a long time.

We had some real cutups in high school, but I don't remember many events worth telling. The Frosty Shop across the street and north of the high school sold soft-serve ice cream, which was new to us then. I don't remember that the school had any food, so we must have been on our own to pack our lunch or go out. Some of us were eating at the Frosty Shop one day when a farmer parked his tractor, pulling a full load of manure, on the high school side of the street. He had apparently come to eat. As we walked back to school on our return trip, Lloyd Tino stopped by the tractor and placed the power takeoff in gear. Lloyd was a farm boy and knew how tractors operated. We did not see or hear about the outcome, but if that farmer did not check his power takeoff gearshift before starting his engine, his load would have immediately spread onto the street and the cars parked behind him.

My sisters remind me that I was given a birthday party at our home during my freshman year, and they never had one. I invited all my old friends as well as my new city and political friends from school. I remember only that we played volleyball in the backyard. Croquette was big then, so I suspect we played that and ate plenty of country food. I'll bet I showed them Elsie the Dirty Pig, too.

Elaine Pollert and Karen Pullen liked my politics at school and became my unofficial campaign managers during my high school years. They would coach me and then bawl me out when I didn't sit up straight on stage. I have not thanked them enough for what they did for my self-image in those years. Another great help to me was Charlie Warner, who faithfully encouraged me in sports.

I took premed courses in high school. A doctor friend said that Latin would be important, so I took that as my language elective for two years. It was difficult for me and not too useful. I was the only boy in the class, so I got babied and received higher grades than I deserved. Typing was my most useful course in high school.

I had most of my required courses done by the middle of my junior year, so I felt I could take FFA, which is where all of my farm friends were. It was an easier course than the premed ones, and it had its own social life. The grading was easier, and it was fun to be able to read farm magazines in class. The citizenship award was given to one student each year, usually a senior. Neil Johnson taught FFA and I know that he was instrumental in my receiving that award in my junior year.

Twyla won the FFA Sweetheart contest in her junior year and received her white jacket and pin, all presented in a nice ceremony on stage. I was in junior college chemistry class during the time of Twyla's ceremony. Mr. Johnson graciously arranged for our college chemistry class to stand at the back doors of the auditorium and watch the presentation to Twyla. This was a big honor for Twyla. Unfortunately, she did not get many of her things out of their old farmhouse when it was abandoned, and that jacket deteriorated with most everything else in the upstairs of that home. Her gold pin was stolen when our Cholla house was broken into in the early 1980s.

Somewhere around my senior year, about the time I started dating Twyla, my folks purchased a used New Yorker Chrysler for me from Stanley Forrest. It was more car than I needed, but gas was about fifteen cents per gallon then. We affectionately named the car "the brown turd," and it served us well through the rest of our school years and into practice. Mr. Emery (Jeff's dad) sold the car for us in about 1963 for fifty dollars, and we split that with him. We bought a smaller Plymouth for three hundred dollars, which I drove until Jeff joined me in practice in 1970. Jeff then found us a 1963 Lincoln Continental which we drove through the air force days until 1975.

The Emery family owned the hardware store in La Salle, as well as a large flying service at the Greeley Airport. Jeff was their son and would eventually attend the same osteopathic school in Des Moines that I did and would join me in practice as a partner.

I had three years of college premed, the first two being at Clarinda Junior College. Farming was not doing well at that time, and the folks did not want me to farm. They wanted me to be any kind of nontraditional doctor, as they didn't trust traditional medicine, for some reason. I can credit Mike Caviness, a counselor in high school, with telling me to "be at least an osteopath" rather than a chiropractor. Money appeared to be short, and junior college was very inexpensive—plus I could stay at home to help and work.

I needed at least a third year of college and some specific courses in order to apply to osteopathic or medical schools. Some hard courses remained for that year, and I transferred to The University of Nebraska at Omaha. Organic chemistry was very difficult for me. I rented a room and daily breakfast from a widow and would drive the Chrysler home each weekend and teach accordion on Saturdays. There were no school activities for me except studying.

Most premed students had four years of college and a degree. I was accepted to COMS (College of Osteopathic Medicine and Surgery) with three years, thanks to Dr. Ford's help, I believe. I had spent as much time as possible with Dr. Ford in Elmo, Missouri, in my premed years. He would allow me to shadow him while he saw patients, and he taught me a lot about medicine and life.

Des Moines COMS was the closest osteopathic or medical school, and I had done everything close to home. I didn't know that one should apply to multiple schools, and I had no backup plan.

I worked for several summers, during high school and early college, at the ASC office (Agriculture Stabilization and Conservation) in Clarinda for one dollar per hour. I was a planimeter operator, which meant measuring crop acres from aerial maps by tracing its borders. At that time the government was buying corn off the market as well as reducing crop acres—all to reduce the supply of corn in order to bring the prices up. I did go to the fields occasionally to measure them by hand with an apparatus that consisted of mainly just a wheel that would roll across the ground to obtain a measurement. One farmer north of town ordered me off his land and threatened to run over me with his tractor. Some farmers didn't appreciate the government's "help."

Mr. Albert Rope was the ASC office administrator at that time, and he was my transportation to and from work. He drove a large Nash car which I just worshipped and enjoyed riding in. I thought it neat that the Nash seats made into a bed with just a flip of two levers. The folks had a Nash for several years and we thought they were great. Twyla got my job at the ASC office after I was gone, and she got paid a dollar twenty-five per hour.

I had started piano lessons sometime in my grade school years, taking from Mr. Schamber and later Mrs. Sunderman. It did not come easily for me, and I distinctly remember Mr. Schamber and myself sitting on the bench at a lesson and both crying.

A group came to Clarinda around that time giving accordion lessons and selling instruments. One would rent the small 12-bass accordion until it was determined whether the student had any promise. They, of course, *all* had promise, and the 120-bass accordions would be purchased. Once the market was maxed out, the crooks would stop lessons and move on to another town and sell more accordions there at their inflated price. My folks purchased a beautiful red 120-bass accordion for four hundred dollars, which, I am sure, was more than we could afford. Their markup on the instruments was at least three- to four-hundred percent. The Midwest is full of attics with slightly used accordions.

Most students did not continue much past the purchase of the expensive instrument, especially when the lessons were no longer available. I did not realize it at the time, but I was not a natural at music, and I advanced just because of hard work. Someone a little more honest did come to town to give lessons and sell more instruments after that first group left, and I continued lessons with that group. Mr. Nuss, the leader of that group, later set up a studio in a hotel room in Red Oak and told me to go teach. I said I couldn't, but he said, "Go ahead, it's easy." I guess by then I'd had enough lessons that I found it easy to teach.

After Mr. Nuss left the area, I continued to teach, as there were plenty of kids with accordions and no teacher. I first taught in homes and later the armory basement, and still later, I had a basement studio on Sixteenth Street across from the Linderman Hotel and the ASC office. I paid Mr. Witthoft (a distant relative) fifteen dollars per month to rent the space. I taught there on Saturdays while in junior college and drove home each weekend from Omaha to give lessons.

The "studio" was a single room about fifteen feet square and painted a heavy yellow–gold, both walls and ceiling. I did some cleaning and painting. Uncle Paul noted that the pipes running across the ceiling were quite ugly and suggested black paint for the ceiling and pipes, which made them hardly show at all. I sawed three boards of decreasing lengths and painted them black, then painted one word on each—accordions, lessons, and music. These were hung vertically, one below another, with small gold chains. I still have two of those boards as a memento. Lee Wagoner found the signs in a pile of boards when they bought our old farm place. He kept them and gave them to Vera to deliver to me.

I sold music with only minimal profit as well as a few accordions, which I marked up one hundred percent. I was to show prospective buyers—the parents—my catalog, with the greatly inflated suggested retail price shown below each instrument. The price that I would pay as a dealer for the accordion was on a separate white sheet, not intended to be seen by the buyer. That is not the way we did it. I actually showed customers my price and told them that theirs would be twice what I paid. No one ever tried to have me reduce the price, as they knew that it was an honest price—especially considering what had gone on before. The accordions were good quality instruments, and I never had any trouble with them that I could not easily fix. I ordered a beautiful gold-and-white accordion for sister Irma one Christmas for one hundred twenty-five dollars, but I soon confiscated it and used it for the rest of my accordion times. It has recently been sent to New Jersey for an eight-hundred-dollar refurbishing. I just love that accordion, as do our kids, so it will be passed on at some time—and hopefully in working condition. Sorry, Irma, I must still get you something else for your 1955 Christmas.

I don't remember any time that I was not paid in full during my business in Clarinda. There were no accounts receivable and no billing. New accordions came by train from Ohio, and it was always so exciting to pick one up. Accordions don't go out of tune and almost nothing goes wrong with them. I taught a maximum of twenty-two students on Saturdays, and we held several recitals. Diane Haxby was my most advanced student, and I turned the business over to her when I left for osteopathic school in Des Moines. Jerome Wagoner had a very nice black accordion, which I lusted after. I should have ordered one like it—it would cost thousands now and was probably a few hundred then.

Dad did a pretty good job of playing the old German-style concertino accordion. A different note was produced when the bellows were closing than when they were opening. We don't know where he learned to play that instrument but doubt that he had any formal lessons. I believe that Dad did play an instrument in a band in Clarinda at one time. Mother played the piano, but never in public and mostly religious songs.

Dad enjoyed entertaining and pulling jokes on people. He embarrassed Mabel Sunderman (my future mother-in-law) once with some fake dog doo-doo and fart-smelling perfume. This happened when Dad and Mabel were teenagers, and the incident nearly derailed *our* wedding some years later. Twyla's Mom and my Dad never did like each other after that joke.

Dad liked to play a joke where he would do multiple measurements on a person with a ruler, supposedly to measure their flexibility. The last measurement was how high the person could lift their knee up on the wall from a kneeling position. He then would ask the person to bark. I don't know how he got anyone to go along with that trick to get to that point. As you can tell, the humor was rather "earthy" but was in keeping with the times, background, and region of the country. Most of Dad's tricks and jokes were thought-out or planned ahead, and he was not spontaneously funny. He would occasionally have a one-liner, usually making fun of someone or of something they had done. Dad's magic shows were always squeaky clean, however.

My folks, as well as others of that area and time, did not appear to like successful people, and could be ruthless in their criticism. They liked to root for the underdog. I believe that some of this was religious influence (root of all evil; eye of the needle; he who carest for the least of these; the first shall be last; etc.). I notice that, even now, Midwest humor points out an individual's failings in a joking way. It is not malicious, however, and well accepted as part of a greeting. The recipient of the joke appeared to enjoy the attention.

Midwest hand waves have their own meaning. Most of these occur when meeting a vehicle or farm equipment on the roads. A slight nod or anemic wave of the hand is just a friendly greeting for someone you probably don't know. A wave with a single index finger raised means that the person is recognized, but not well known. A definite acquaintance would get a hearty wave with a pointing of the index finger.

Dad would go to Clarinda or Shenandoah and hire someone for the season or longer to help with the farm work. These men would agree to live in our house as part of their pay. A favorite joke of Dad's would be to drive up to the most dilapidated farm place that he could find on the way home and say, "Here we are." I did this same scenario to Nathan (our daughter Valerie's husband) in regard to wedding planning. Nathan did not know me well at all but knew that we had done much wedding planning. Nathan was up from Tucson and we drove them around Phoenix to finalize plans. I drove up to the most dilapidated motel that I could find on Van Buren Street in the red-light district and said, "Here we are—the wedding site." Poor Nathan was not used to jokes like that, and it was almost too much for him.

Ivan Otte was a cousin of Dad's who lived about a mile west of us. Ivan loved to have fun also, and he and Maxine were part of our social circle. There are many funny stories about Ivan—it was almost like there was a cloud over him sometimes. One time, Ivan and Dad and Ralph Wagoner made a trip to Valentine, Nebraska, to buy cattle. Now, Ralph was the nicest person you could imagine, but he could not pronounce certain sounds, probably due to the genetic absence of some tongue or facial muscle. The three men stopped at a restaurant for supper on the way home. Ivan went in ahead of the other two and talked with the owner of the restaurant. Ivan told him that he and Orval were transporting a mental patient and that that third person could have only an egg salad sandwich—no matter what he ordered. Poor Ralph tried and tried, with his garbled speech, to order a steak like the other two but all he got was egg salad. This story generated many good, loving laughs back home. Ralph loved the story as much as anyone. The episode may have worked so well because Clarinda, at that time, had a two-thousand-patient state mental health facility.

One of Dad's favorite untrue stories was to tell about when the two hired men caught a stray dog, of which there were plenty, dragged the animal to the gas pump, and filled the dog full of gasoline. That dog then took off running around the farmstead twice, came back to the pump, jumped about six feet high, and fell down to the ground. The subject being told the story would then usually ask if the dog was dead. The answer would be, "No, he ran out of gas."

Being on a farm, we always had a farm dog—but only one at a time. We went through lots of dogs, as our philosophy was that the animals were there to serve us. Neighbors would shoot neighbor's dogs if that dog were chasing cattle—and that seemed to be almost expected.

I enjoy telling animal stories of the farm to some of the local animal lovers of today who will spend any amount of money on the welfare of their pets. They talk about spending sixteen hundred dollars on a knee replacement for their little dog and then worry because the animal has three more legs. I tell them that I can take care of their problem for a penny, like we used to do on the farm—meaning a .22 caliber bullet. I like to brag about how useful the farm dogs were to us, and at no expense. I don't remember a vet bill for the dog—or ever buying a bag of food for the dog. They just ate scraps from our table or whatever they could catch.

A lady asked once what we did with our farm dog when we went on vacation. I told her that we shot the dog when we left, and another stray would show up when we returned home. That did not go over well in that crowd at all, so I tell that story often now, just to see the responses. I don't believe that we ever did shoot our dog, but it had been done by some in those times. I didn't tell the lady that we never took vacations, either. I believe that we were comfortable with using the animals that way because the Bible supposedly says something about the animals being there to serve us.

There were plenty of *true* animal stories that would end one in jail now. Some of our dogs were good hunting dogs, but most were mutts of no known breed and had come from other farms. In order to keep from being overrun with dogs or cats born on one's farm, it was common for farmers to take the extra animals far from home and turn them loose—or, to put the newborns in a gunny sack, tie it shut, and throw it into a pond.

We stored corn on the cob in a large corncrib in the days before combines. It was always a big day when the corn sheller would come. It was a specially made truck where the ear corn would fall or be shoveled into a large spout on the back and then the machine would separate the corn from the cobs. The corn could then be fed or sold, and the cobs used for heating, wiping, or discarding to the ditch. All the mice that were in that corn would suddenly be homeless and running around. At one age, it was sport to catch the mice and kill them. The number of rodents would be too many mice for our farm cats to handle on that day. Sometimes I would store the mice in my pockets until I could climb down from a high place. I can still feel them biting through the fabric.

Ivan Otte once accidentally burned down their outhouse, with himself in it. Our Walther League (a young people's church organization) presented a stage play doing "This is Your Life" episodes on various members of the congregation. We had an outhouse on stage with smoke pouring out, and eventually "Ivan" running out, pulling up his pants and yelling, "Maxine, we're going to lose it."

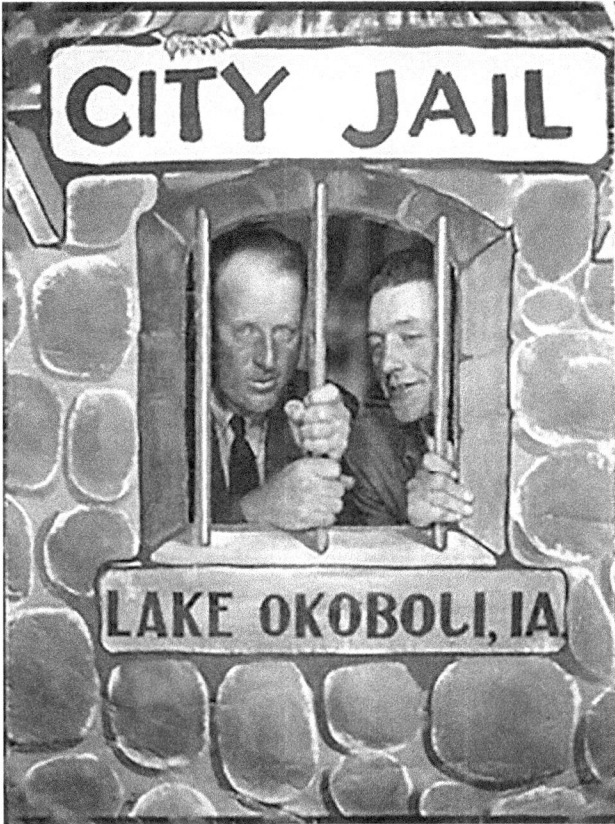

My dad (Orval Otte) and Ivan Otte (Dad's first cousin and neighbor), would do most anything for a laugh. Ivan, who smoked, once burned down their outhouse with him in it—not intending for it to be a laugh.

I don't remember how we showed this, but Ivan had at least one other really bad day. There was a real aggressive and troublesome tomcat that had been keeping him awake at night and also impregnating his domestic cats. Ivan had decided to shoot the tomcat with his shotgun, but he missed, and the cat ran into the culvert at the entrance to the farm. There was a trickle of water running through the tube, so Ivan got the bright idea of floating some gasoline on the water and lighting it. The gasoline naturally soaked very well into the cat's fur, just as Ivan had hoped. He lit the floating gasoline "fuse" and, of course, the cat was a ball of fire when he ran out of the tube—straight for the hog house. Ivan had planned to shoot the cat upon its exit, but again, he missed—probably because of the speed of the target. Ivan had just bedded the hog house down with fresh straw, which easily became a large blaze, and they lost the hog house too. We assume that the cat perished in the fire.

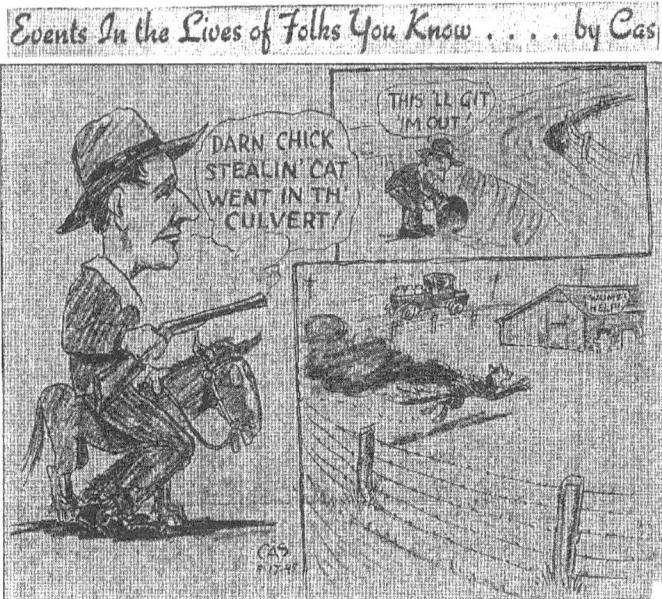

Events In the Lives of Folks You Know . . . . by Cas

Ivan Otte had a problem. A tomcat was keeping them awake at night and was stealing his chickens. As you know, farmers can fix about anything with gasoline, duct tape, barbed wire, and a shotgun. Ivan missed with his first shot from the 410 and the cat ran into the culvert under the entrance to his farm place. He tried everything to get that cat to leave the culvert so he could get another shot. There was a trickle of water running through that tube, so it seemed reasonable to Ivan to pour some gasoline on the water and let it soak into the cat's fur. He then lit the gasoline trickle and the fire went right to the cat. The animal shot out on fire and ran faster than ever. Ivan missed the second shot also and the cat ran right to his hog house which contained his sows and new pigs and a fresh batch of straw. I don't remember what happened to the hog house or the cat, but Ivan really had a bad day.

The local paper, The Clarinda Herald Journal, was a biweekly publication and held a much higher importance in those early times, having no competition from other media as we have now. Mr. Caswell was its editor and a very good cartoonist as well. He would draw a cartoon on the front page each week, depicting some funny or stupid thing done by a local person. I know that both of these episodes involving Ivan were characterized in that way. I believe that Dad and Grandpa were also shown in his cartoons at different times but can't remember what for.

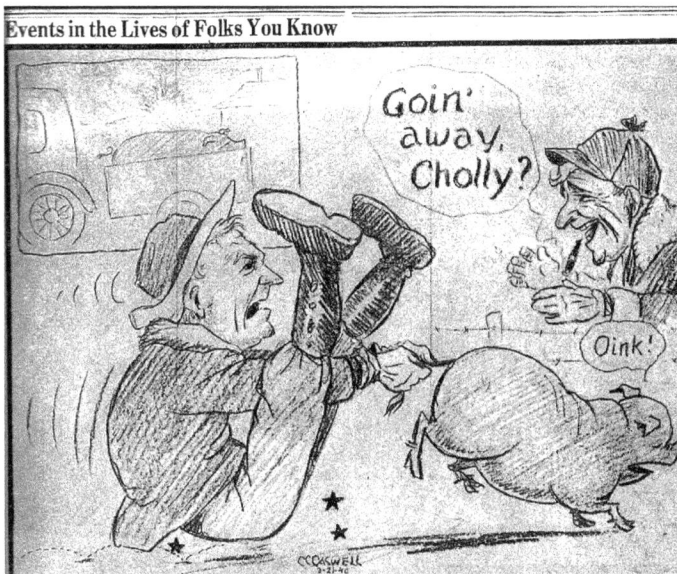

The Clarinda Herald Journal came twice weekly and the editor was Caswell. For years he would do a drawing or caricature of something stupid or funny that happened that week to someone in the Clarinda area. His drawings became so well known that locals would watch for happenings and "tattle" to Caswell. This one was my grandfather Charlie who butchered pigs for the County Home.

Several church happenings during this time period are worth telling. The old church (which looked like the current Bethesda church) had no air conditioning. One of the portly members decided to open a side window during the sermon one Sunday. He wore a belt with no suspenders, and when he reached up to open the window, his pants dropped to his ankles. Being in church, the women all tried to look away quickly and act like no one saw.

The local Lutheran custom was to stand immediately after the "Amen" at the close of the sermon. The older grade school kids were allowed to sit in the balcony. Willard Herzberg had fallen asleep one Sunday and the person behind him whispered a loud amen in his ear. Willard, thinking that the sermon had ended, stood bolt upright and then noticed that he was the only one standing during the sermon. Willard could catch flies in school with his hands while the rest of us watched, amazed at his skill. He claimed that flies take off backward, so he aims the hand sweep behind where the fly was sitting.

The youngest school-age children had to sit downstairs in the front row of the congregation. Those a little older would be in the second row. One Sunday Pastor Kreutz paused his sermon because some girls in one of those rows were talking or showing billfolds to each other. I won't mention names, because all of you may know these perpetrators, but it was very embarrassing for them. Some of them still talk a lot.

Family magic shows have been a part of our lives as long as I can remember. I really don't know why Dad had such a passion for magic or how he got started, but I believe he was self-taught. The upper left drawer of the buffet always contained an assortment of joke and small magic items. The folks had quite a lot of larger magic items for their stage magic shows—as well as a canary or two. Dad could easily have done a two-hour magic show without any repeats, and his shows were pure rapid-fire tricks without much patter. Many of the magicians of that time would do only a few tricks in an hour because of all their talking and showmanship. Dad's tricks were pretty well "canned" with a few really clean 1940s jokes. He did lots of shows through the years at churches, fairs, 4-H and farm events, and for business meetings. His fee was whatever the organization could afford, but often in the twenty-five-dollar range. The family show traveled a few hundred miles from home in the four-state area. He probably averaged one show per week for thirty or forty years. They incorporated the family when we were available and adjusted as we aged and left home. A magic show trumped any other event, and I don't remember missing any of the shows while we were at home. About once per week, we would do chores early and drive off to do our show. Our audiences would usually be several hundred people.

Mom was not a natural performer, so she did as little as possible onstage, but she did support Dad backstage. She would load the rabbits and canaries into the tricks, load the milk into the milk tricks, and generally keep things moving and orderly backstage. Mom and Dad had a comedic mind-reading act, which involved the audience and was really quite funny. I would not be embarrassed to do that act, even now.

Irma and Vera helped backstage, and they also did a balancing act and sang. They were part of a comedy levitation act, which was very believable—until the secret was revealed. Ruth, being the smallest then, could fit into some tight quarters. Dad actually built a small church on stage and, to the song of "Let's Go to Church Next Sunday Morning," Ruth would raise the roof and come out. This was often the finale.

Dad would bake a cake on stage and the result would be a rabbit or two in the pan. He had tricks with lit candles; a lit lightbulb that would have a canary in it; various tricks with large cards; rope tricks; tricks with large rings; and sponges and bottle tricks. Each trick would have a surprise or comical ending, and Dad seldom screwed up. He involved the audience in quite a few parts of the act, and that was always well received.

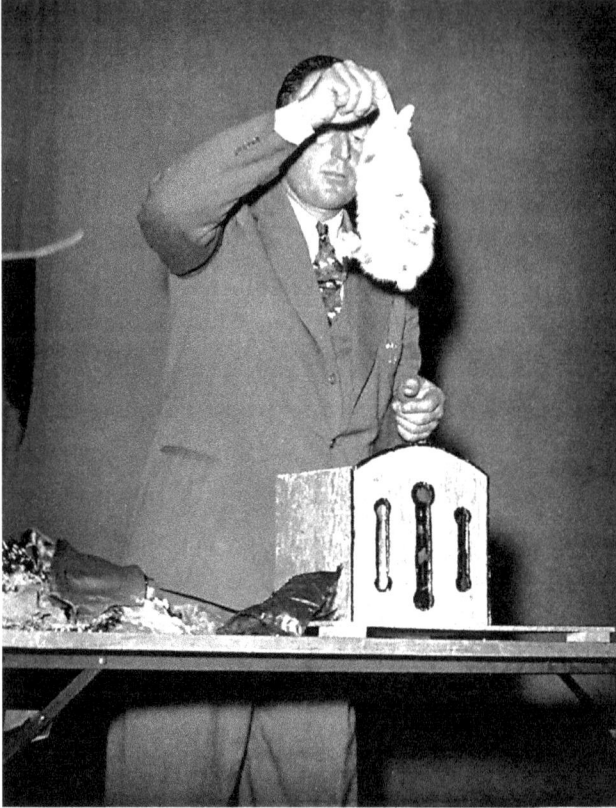

Dad did the magic and Mom kept things "loaded" and cleaned
up. She didn't like being on stage. Dad has produced a rabbit
from a box.

Dad had large farmer's hands with calluses, so did not attempt to
work with any of the smaller items that would require dexterity. I,
therefore, did the work with cards, thimbles, and some of the small
ropes. I played an accordion solo at some point during each show and
would play background music for some of the tricks.

Our family could not afford to eat out, but a banquet often
preceded our performance, so we experienced plenty of good food
associated with the shows. My sisters and I still get along very well,
and I attribute that to having a common purpose and activities while
we were growing up.

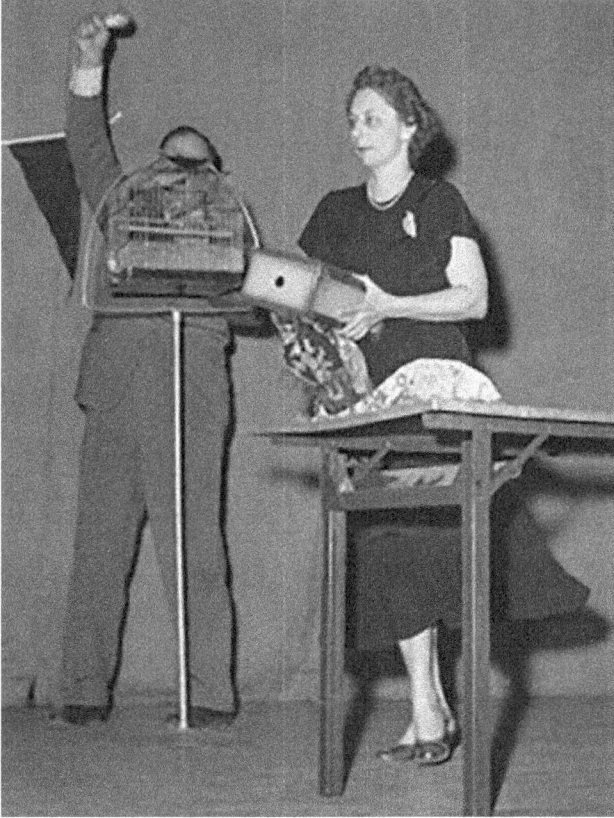

Here Dad has a canary in a light bulb

Dad tried to keep up and learn new tricks. He was a regular subscriber to the "Tops" magazine and attended the Abbott Magic Conventions in Colon, Michigan. The folks enjoyed those conventions very much and would meet some famous performers there. Harry Blackstone (possibly the world's greatest magician of the time) is buried in Colon and we have been there to visit his grave. Our family attended one of Blackstone's last shows in Omaha on a very bad icy night. We hung around after the show and were able to talk with him, and I actually drove him to his hotel. I was very worried about driving on the ice and being responsible for such an important person. He signed my program from the show and died soon afterward, but at least not from my driving. I wish I had kept that signed program.

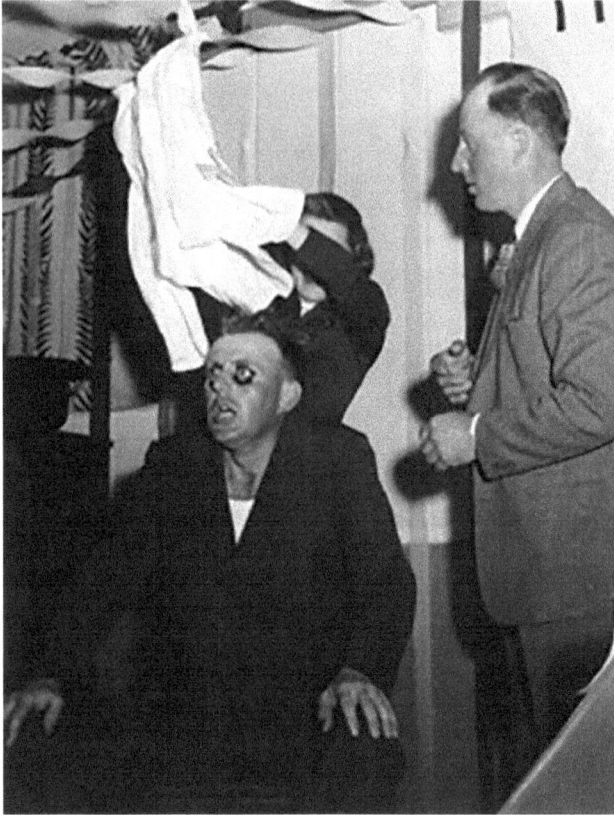

Dad removing a shirt from Herb Rope after he came to the stage with shirt, coat, and tie on. The tie was cut up and then reappeared at the end.

The folks were gone out of state for a week sometime while I was in high school and the other three girls were in grade school or early high school. We received a call to do a magic program on short notice for a county fair in Missouri—their planned program probably cancelled at the last minute. We kids had all been doing our parts of the magic program, and I could do most of the larger tricks, so we decided to take the program all by ourselves. It was an outdoor program, which presents more problems with audience control. The show was a catastrophe, and we almost got booed off the stage. The folks couldn't believe that we had taken that job.

The folks continued to do shows even after the kids were out of the house. Their magic props have now been divided between Irma, Vera, Ruth, and me. It is hard to part with items that were such a long-term part of our family history, but none of us are doing magic shows. I do a little magic about once per year now, mostly with the grandchildren. Maybe that will occur more often or maybe some of them will take an interest in the hobby or profession.

On another subject entirely, we had a family friend from a small town nearby in South Dakota. "Doc" had been a family friend since the '30s or '40s. His story is very interesting and intriguing, and I would guess that I know less than one percent of it. He was well revered and called "doctor" by most who knew him. The only ones to call him by his first name were some of the locals. He had no doctorate, however, and I doubt he held a college or even a high school diploma. He told us once that he had attended a six-week course at a masseur school in Chicago, and I wish I had asked more questions about his training. He had an unusual ability to learn from experience and to influence people. He said that he learned much from catching small animals as a child and dislocating and then relocating (reducing) their joints. His "treatments," however, did not involve anything that traumatic, and I don't know of him ever reducing a joint in practice.

He claimed to be able to diagnose and treat by palpating and rubbing areas of the neck and back. He could feel areas of local muscle spasm (which is very easy to do with a little experience) and could tell the patient which areas were painful to the touch. Rubbing the tenderness out of these areas certainly relieved the local discomfort, but he insinuated that this would diagnose and relieve conditions or illness in other body organs. He had a quiet way about him that caused the patient to think that "Doc" was holding back and struggling with how much to reveal to the individual—for the patient's own good. He had a unique ability to observe and listen carefully and then turn that information into "new findings" that would amaze the patient. I truly don't believe that he was trying to be dishonest, merely maximizing the confidence that the patient would have in him. We understand now the importance of the patient's confidence in treatment. The benefits of massage are also now being recognized and accepted—to the tune of about eighty dollars per hour in many spas. The idea of diagnosing from structural findings is not entirely out of line and is a still a part of osteopathic teachings. Doc was way ahead of his time and didn't know it. He helped many people, and during most of his years, charged only one dollar per treatment. He had been married, and his wife died of cancer before my memories of him.

I believe our family was introduced to Doc by Uncle Ed and Aunt Lena, who resided at Wessington Springs, South Dakota. They were very much new frontier farmers who had moved to Dakota during the depression in an attempt to make a better living. They survived on a small farm in the dust bowl days from being very frugal, I suspect. They likely did not have much fun, as we think of fun. They would have looked a lot like the Grant Wood painting "American Gothic." Their house was small, and the land was flat and always seemed dry. We visited them on most of our trips to Dakota, as they were only eighty miles from the town where Doc was. I remember sleeping upstairs in an attic-like room on a soft featherbed.

Uncle Ed may have been a little compulsive. Birthday cards were very important to him, and he would keep them in the exact order in which they had arrived. They came to one of the annual Goecker Christmas gatherings at Uncle Otto's or at Emmy and Melie's in Yorktown. I thought it would be a good joke to tease Uncle Ed about South Dakota crops. I took in two pans of ear corn from the crib and labeled the pans as Iowa corn and South Dakota corn. I, of course, picked out the best ears for the Iowa pan and nubbins for the Dakota pan. I then showed the two pans around to everyone at the party, but Uncle Ed did not even crack a smile, and I shouldn't have done that.

Anyway, the story was that Aunt Lena was gored badly by a bull at some early time and had some disabilities from that. She limped badly, so I assume she had a hip injury. She also had vitiligo, just like Michael Jackson, and blamed that on the bull as well. They had heard of Doc, so they visited him sometime in the late 1930s and did get relief for Aunt Lena. For that reason, my grandparents and parents started going to Doc. My mother had a back condition that was supposedly leading toward surgery and got either relief or a cure from Doc. It was almost three hundred miles to Doc's place from Clarinda, which was quite a trip in the 1930s and '40s, but the trip was made almost yearly for thirty years. He promised to fix most anything and claimed he had worked with Sister Kenny and could stop polio—so we had little fear of that disease. There were not a lot of places to stay in the small town about five miles from Doc's farm, so the folks made friends with some of Doc's neighbors, and we stayed with them. Grandpa Otte and I went alone once in the early days of our visits to Doc and stayed in a hotel room in the small town—a room that had only one door and no windows. I hope we paid Doc's neighbors with whom we stayed (the Andersons and Pearsons), but I really don't know. Later on, we stayed with Doc himself in his country house on the farm. Mom would do some cooking and household duties, and I'm sure Doc appreciated the good food.

We would look out in the mornings and see twenty or thirty cars loaded with patients parked in his driveway. Remember that this all took place on a farmstead. There was no system, but the patients seemed to keep track of who was next, and I don't remember ever having any problem. We have pictures of those cars at sunup on many days. People would wait in their cars and would come into the house to wait as their turn approached. Doc originally gave his treatments in his bedroom in the front of his house. He would get up, eat something, make his bed, set up a straight chair in the bedroom and open the front door to start the day. The chair was the only prop that he needed. He would stand or sit behind the patient and rub their neck and back in short circular motions. Each treatment would last about five minutes, and he would do over a hundred treatments on many days.

With the number of patients Doc saw, up to a hundred some days, one might expect there to be some unending days. That never happened. People would quit coming, and we were always out of people by five, or no later than seven p.m. Folks would quit coming late in the day out of respect for quitting time, even though we had no hours posted. I don't remember anyone ever coming to the door after we had gone to the house. People always paid, and Doc would stuff the bills into his pocket. I don't know what happened then, as we never visited a bank.

When we did stay with Doc, we would use his upstairs bedrooms. Any time that we would come downstairs, the small living and dining rooms would be packed with patients awaiting their turns. We would each receive a treatment each day, usually at the end of his day— which could be late. There was no system that I know of to control the daily patient load. Perhaps people went on if they saw too many cars ahead of them. The setting was remarkably simple.

Dad and Uncle Paul say that in later years, they built a small clinic for Doc in the trees just west of his house and lane. I remember it being a simple white stucco building with one larger waiting room and one small treatment room. I believe it was heated with one potbelly stove in the waiting room which, I'm sure, was run by the patients. The treatment room must have been heated passively, because the door opened so often.

Doc never took vacation, but he did come to visit the folks several times. Dad would arrange a load of patients for him to see while there, and I remember our house being full of people at those times. There were a lot of people from the Clarinda area who had made sojourns to see Doc in Dakota and it was a chance for them to avoid a long trip.

Doc drove new Chrysler New Yorkers and that would have been his only excess. When he had too much cash he would buy another farm, so he had four farms. Everything was done in cash, and I don't know that he had a checking account.

I wanted badly to learn Doc's treatment methods, so I spent at least the summer of 1958 with him—that was between premed and osteopathic school. I was with him every day with every patient. He would have me do a few things with the patients, but basically, I observed. There was really no scientific learning, but I learned much about communication skills. The treatments were basically to find the tender spots and rub them until not tender. I don't want to minimize his skills and technique, as they were successful and should be used more. Given the way doctors have to rush now, they can't or don't take time for this type of treatment. It has been relegated to physical therapy and become very expensive. Massage can give great relief to patients with musculoskeletal pain and for stress-related complaints. I used Doc's techniques frequently in my ten years of general practice, but less so in the ER.

Doc and I lived like bachelors during the summer or two I was with him and must have eaten lots of peanut butter. I don't remember eating out much at all. His town, five miles away, had only a few bars in it. Doc was truly on a farm. There were no doctors of any kind in the area, and probably none any closer than forty miles away. No regulation of nontraditional doctors existed then and probably not now, either.

The Ortmans were a chiropractic family with a large, well-known clinic in Canistota, South Dakota. Now Doc did not approve of the Ortmans, but the clinic was on the way to Doc's and was interesting to see. Doc did not know we stopped there. This clinic was kind of the Mayo Clinic of chiropractic, at least locally. The Ortmans seemed to own the town. Believers would come to Canistota and stay a week to receive treatments. There was not a lot to do in the town, but one painter named Pletan had a shop on the main street. He would entertain with his paintings (which he sold) and always had a crowd. Mr. Pletan drank a lot, or at least acted like he did. It took him only five to ten minutes to finish a beautiful picture. He would be nearly done with a picture when he would "slip" and make a big ugly line across the painting—and would then turn that line into a tree or something appropriate to the drawing. I remember that Dad did some magic for the crowd at times, and we would receive pictures in payment.

The only bathroom in Doc's house was a single commode out in the open in the basement. It was a dark and somewhat damp basement, and one had to pass by a full skeleton in the hallway to reach that commode. I hated going down into that basement, but that was the only stool in the house. Come to think of it, what *did* all those patients do for a bathroom, as there was none other, and I know that they didn't go down that basement. A small red barn sat at the south end of the drive, and I suspect that was heavily used for all those years. That ground should be growing some good crops by now. I'm sure that there were no provisions for the disabled, either. I don't remember a bathroom, even in the clinic.

There was one day that Doc needed to pay for something with eight hundred dollars, so he went to the closet and got a shoebox full of money to pay that bill. Uncle Paul stayed at Doc's house once. He said that a drawer was ajar in their bedroom and upon pulling the drawer out to close it, he noted that it was full of cash. He says that naturally, he looked in the other drawers then and found they were full of money too. Now, Uncle Paul is known for telling some very believable tall stories. I cannot confirm his tale, but it makes a good story. It would not have been my nature, however, to look in drawers unless I had a reason to do so. I probably lived out of a suitcase when I stayed with Doc. I borrowed eight hundred dollars from him for my schooling in Des Moines and repaid him in cash soon after Twyla and I were married.

The folks and Uncle Paul's family worshipped the ground that Doc walked on. Doc became interested in a product called ISO–Mite in the mid '50s, and he planned for Dad to be the distributor for Iowa and

Uncle Paul for Missouri and Nebraska. The product was an engine or transmission additive which was a chemical combination of copper and lead. The product, when added to an engine, was to "plate out" in the opposing parts of the engine. It was to fill the voids and actually rebuild an old engine to new tolerances. The lead was to lubricate, while the copper was to transfer heat away from the friction areas more effectively than other metals. It was said to stop use of oil and smoking of the engine and greatly improve mileage. The longer the product was used, the more benefit. It came suspended in oil in small cans for engines and in grease for use in any areas where grease would be used. It was also available in quarts of a synthetic oil to be used in place of petroleum products. Uncle Paul suspended some of the crystals in a wax and made ISO–Mite pills for addition to engines. A favorite demonstration was to show how long a small engine which had been "treated" could be run without oil. Dad held a demonstration on one of Lee Wagoner's tractors one cold day with many in attendance, but the gasoline use was decreased by only about five percent. Theoretically, that would improve more with time.

Several of Doc's friends from California came to his hometown to get the project started. Doc intended to manufacture the product in his hometown and actually laid footings for the factory downtown. The folks and Uncle Paul's were each "drop-shipped" five thousand dollars' worth of ISO–Mite to get their distributorships started. We stored it in our garage, and I went out to look at it every day. It seemed like a magic product and a sure thing. I was a high school kid at the time and actually wanted Dad to sell the farm and dedicate full time to the Iowa distributorship.

I still believe that ISO–Mite was a good product, but there was one thing that stopped the project in its tracks—the IRS. Doc had always done everything by cash, so the IRS didn't know that he existed until he started throwing money around for the ISO–Mite business. The IRS took his farms and any other assets they could find and forced him into bankruptcy. Some of Doc's neighbors bought the farms and held them for him as they knew that he would recover. This, of course, stopped all of the ISO–Mite Midwest division.

Uncle Paul claims he was waiting in the clinic the day the two young IRS agents came to do their initial questioning of Doc. He says the agents wanted a witness, so Doc asked Paul to come into the treatment room for the interview. He said the agents had been very polite and waited their turn. They asked Doc how he paid for his Chrysler and Doc said, "Oh, I just saved up for it." When asked how he could afford the farms, he said, "Oh, they kind of paid for themselves." The agents agreed to let Doc finish his patients for the day and said they would be back at ten o'clock the next morning. Uncle Paul claims that the two friends from California helped Doc bury cream cans full of money that night. Uncle Paul also claims that Doc spent several years in prison, but I don't believe that happened.

Doc did recover quickly, but never did get to do the ISO–Mite business that he had hoped. He raised his treatment price from one dollar to three dollars after that. His business was still mostly cash. The IRS had a log book for patients to sign, but I believe few signed that. It wasn't long before he had his farms back, and he continued to treat patients as long as his health allowed.

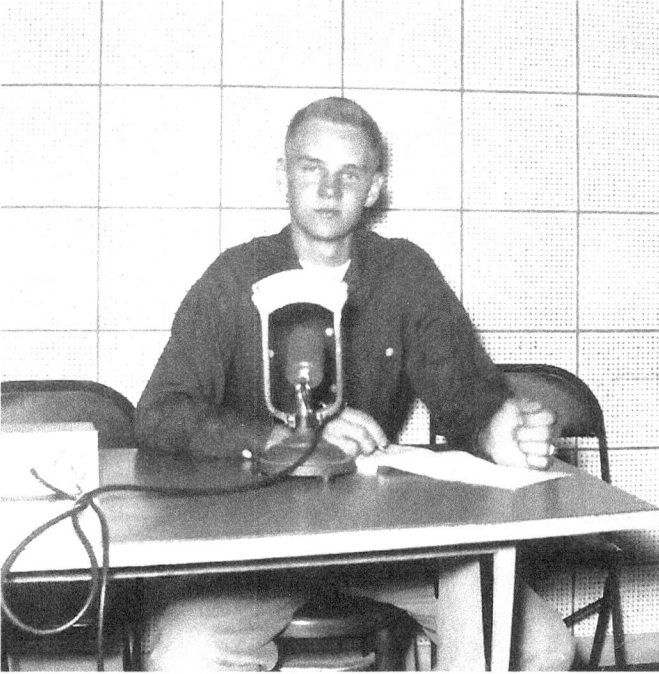

I was organizer and interviewer/introducer for the Clarinda
segment of The Teen Talent Show on KFNF.

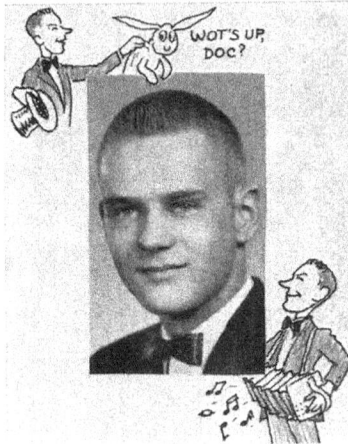

I had a hundred of these printed in my senior year and sent
most of them out. There were no responses.

Chapter Three

Premed Years

I came to a fork in the road of my life sometime in the early 1950s in regard to my profession. I could either attend the Air Force Academy or go into some type of healing profession. Given the fascination our families had with alternative healing, my path became the latter. Two of our family doctors had been osteopaths, and a high school counselor said, "At least be an osteopath." In retrospect, my extreme interest in flying (specifically fighters) would seem to indicate that the academy would have been a good choice and a life-changing decision. Aunt Tina had suggested the academy and was willing to help with the political appointment. I believe we just didn't think it possible for me to get into the academy, and the application process must have terminated that option out of fear of the unknown.

High school courses were all geared toward premed, including my two years of Latin. I was the only male in the class, but still didn't love the subject. The doctor friend who suggested I take Latin said it would help in the naming of bones, but I didn't find it useful, and it may have even misled me at times. As it turns out, Spanish would have been more helpful, but I refuse to learn that now, as we speak English in this country.

The most useful class from high school turned out to be typing. From the medical preparatory standpoint, high school was uneventful, except that I did miss out on some of the more fun classes that my friends took. I always felt the subtle pressure to do well in the more difficult classes recommended for premed. Some of the premed classes still appear to me to have been useless. As early students, we have no experience to know what is going to be useful, so we study everything suggested. I understand the "weeding out" of some who might not be able to handle the curriculum, but I feel that the weeding is efficient for the admission committees and very unfair to the individual and to the future of medicine.

Medical and osteopathic schools in the 1950s required a minimum of three years college preadmission. Because of cost, I did the first two of those years at Clarinda Junior College. At that time the college was in the high school building and seemed like a continuation of high school. My third year was at the University of Omaha. This allowed me to continue to help on the farm and to continue my accordion teaching business. I commuted to Omaha each Monday morning and returned home each Friday evening. We rented a room for the weekdays from Mrs. Grosse, about one mile from the university. Kitchen privileges were available each evening so I could cook something for the evening meal—usually Lipton's chicken noodle soup, a typical low-budget college meal. I participated in no school or social activities and only studied. Even during the year in Omaha, my Saturday was filled with ten hours of teaching accordion at my studio in Clarinda. Any spare time in those last two or three summers was spent working on the farm or traveling to Elmo, Missouri, to observe Dr. Ford in his practice. I also traveled to South Dakota during parts of the last two summers to observe our doctor friend in his practice.

Chapter Four

Osteopathic School

1958-1962

The fall of 1958 found me attending The College of Osteopathic Medicine and Surgery (COMS) in Des Moines, Iowa. I believe Dr. Ford pulled some strings to get me into COMS, as I had only three years of college and a borderline organic chemistry grade. COMS was the medical school closest to home, and the school from which several of our family doctors had graduated. I did not know that most premed students applied to multiple schools for admission. I remember driving by myself once to The University of Iowa to investigate and apply to the medical school there. Seeing the grandeur of the complex was too much. I didn't even get out of the car and just drove back home. The folks were not at all supportive of that University of Iowa effort, as they had a strong preference for osteopathy, and besides, I had no confidence or feeling that I deserved the opulent surroundings I'd seen at U of I.

Fortunately, my girlfriend (and later wife) Twyla Sunderman started a three-year nursing program in Des Moines at Iowa Lutheran at the same time I started medical school, in 1958. We had no money, and Twyla's folks paid none of her tuition. Twyla was able to cover her expenses by working extra as a student nurse for a dollar per hour.

My tuition was an incredible eight hundred dollars for the first year, and Dad and Mom somehow came up with that, plus money for my living expenses. It was out of the question to continue the accordion business in Des Moines. I tried to work nights at the Des Moines Club, but was unable to continue due to the heavy class load. Some of the osteopathic students were able to make twenty-five dollars per night working at mortuaries. This involved mostly sitting up with bodies in caskets and would allow considerable study time, but this did not appeal to me.

The physical COMS school building was a five-story red brick structure occupying about a half block on Sixth Avenue in Des Moines, just north of downtown and near Veteran's Auditorium. The building housed multiple classrooms and labs, as well as the clinic where we saw our first patients in our junior and senior years. Buck's Coffee Shop was in the northeast corner on the main floor. This was a popular spot to congregate between and after classes, and was the only spot, besides. We had little time between classes, as students spent about thirty classroom hours (forty actual hours) per week in classes or labs. Fifteen hours was a common load for a premed curriculum. The amount of homework always exceeded the time available to do it.

Osteopathy was not well accepted at that time, so we felt pressure to always try to do it better. We experienced a lot of stress with our attempts to be accepted into mainstream medicine, and we worked hard to do the right things—socially, politically, and medically. One weekend we students painted the entire red brick exterior of the facility white, which enhanced its appearance somewhat. The original building is now gone, and the school has moved to a much nicer facility on Grand Avenue.

The school is now named Des Moines University, and at this time the tuition is in the thirty-five-thousand-dollar range per year. The name of the school has changed frequently through the years, and originally was called Still College after the originator of osteopathy. Across the street from the school was the very small twenty- to thirty-bed Still Hospital. Osteopaths were not yet accepted on staffs of medical hospitals, so they had to support their own hospitals.

Freshmen were required to purchase all their supplies—their books, a real skull, a plastic spine, and a microscope. All these school expenses had to be difficult for the folks to pay for, as we were living partially on money borrowed against the farm. It also took Twyla and me ten years to pay back the ten thousand dollars that we figured we owed for the osteopathic schooling. I'm sure the amount should have been much more, considering the interest the folks had to pay on that money.

We had to wear shirt, tie, and coat or lab jacket at school. I wore the same grey-striped jacket throughout most of the years. The courses were well taught and quite difficult. We osteopaths would eventually have to pass the same basic science and licensing tests as the MDs in most states. By today's standards, not much was done to make efficient use of the students' time. We took notes by hand.

I remember smoking circular drums on a physiograph machine that allowed a needle to record the movement of frog muscles while the drum rotated. The drum would be blackened by smoke, then we'd attach a frog's muscle to a needle to record the actions of the muscle when we exposed it to various chemicals while the drums rotated. We had no way to record those actions, which hardly justified the experiments due to the inefficiency of the methods.

We were given tests in one subject or another almost every day. Seven of us from the Iota Tau Sigma fraternity became study pals, even though I still spent much time on my own in study. The seven of us would take furious notes in class, and we'd all take our turn to gather up these notes and type up a synopsis for distribution to the other six the next day. I'd usually get no sleep on my night to type. My typewriter could make three carbon copies at a time, so I needed to type everything twice to get seven copies. John had helped me buy a used portable typewriter for twenty-five dollars, and I wish now I had kept it. We felt that our system gave us an edge, as some of the professors were extremely regimented and thought that their lectures were much more important than the texts. Thus, we could expect almost all questions to be pulled from the class notes. It was an ego thing with the professors, but we had to deal with it. The fraternities had libraries that held the tests from prior years, and these were invaluable due to the fact that some professors repeated prior tests. A sad side note is that within ten years of graduation, three of the seven in my study group were dead—by suicide, rectal carcinoma, and seminoma.

Out of approximately sixty-eight students in our class, fifty percent were Jewish. Neither of the two female students finished. Class voting was often along Jewish vs. Gentile lines. I had no idea what a fraternity was, but I joined the ITS fraternity. We had the summer off between our first and second years, and that was our last time away. I used most of that summer to be with our "doctor friend" in South Dakota.

The campus provided no housing, so we had to find our own. Two of the other fraternities did have houses. I do best when I study alone, so I would not have done well living in a frat house. I rented an attic room on the third floor of the Henkel Accordion studio, about two miles north of the school on Sixth Avenue. One tends to gravitate to what they know, and I at least knew the Henkels because I had taken a few accordion lessons from them. The room was quite small and required climbing two flights of stairs, but it was a place to hole up and study, which I did almost constantly. The room was literally in the gables of the house, and I could only stand up in the middle of it. I must have rented the room without the folks' input, as I remember how horrified Mom was when she finally came to Des Moines to see my living situation. The room was clean, but much of the time it was cold, so I just wore more clothes. Broadlawns County Hospital sat somewhere north of where I was living, but I never did see it. Sixth Avenue must have been a main artery to that hospital, as ambulances roared by under my window with sirens screaming, twenty-four hours a day. I was so jealous that those MD interns at the county hospital were getting all of that experience. I was still four years away from being an intern, but I knew that the internships available to me at that time would not be getting a high volume of critically sick or injured patients. I really wanted to be a general doctor able to take care of anything that came my way. It took fifteen years, but the Kansas City residency did accomplish that.

Two of my school friends came to study one night, and John Nelson, from Des Moines, insisted that I rent a room from his mother and live with them. I did that for the rest of that first year and got a good breakfast and evening meal each day. I hope that we paid them enough, but money was tight, and I suspect that our rent was low. I study best by myself, however, so I made solo arrangements for the second year.

I needed to find a solo room and wanted to find one in a nice area. To do this, I did as I had done before—find an area of town that I liked and go door to door, even though rooms were not advertised. My first stop was at the home of Mrs. Hicks on Thompson Avenue, about one mile north of Lutheran Hospital where Twyla was in nursing school, and three miles from my school. Fortunately, Mrs. Hicks's adult son was there when I stopped. He was helping his mother put up storm windows on her Tudor-style house. His name was also Carl, and he liked me, so he and his mother agreed to provide a room and one meal per day for fifteen dollars per week. Mrs. Hicks was a widow and seemed to appreciate having someone around. Her evening meals were excellent, much like I was accustomed to, and I stayed at this home for the rest of my time in Des Moines. Twyla moved in after we were married, and that room was our first home. Twyla lived there with me for three months.

For the three months of summer after my junior year and the first six months of my senior year, I saw clinic patients and continued building a clinic practice. The last six months of my senior year consisted of a couple of three-month externships out of town. We left Mrs. Hicks's home at the halfway mark of my senior year.

Twyla started nursing school at Iowa Lutheran in 1958, so we both had left home and gone to Des Moines in the same year. We dated during the next three years but had no money. Twyla worked at Iowa Lutheran Hospital for a dollar per hour during her last two years. We shared rides and expenses on our infrequent visits to Clarinda. Twyla's schooling lasted three years, and we married soon after she graduated in 1961, so were married during my senior year.

Twyla reminds me that we often studied at Thompson Park near Mrs. Hicks's home, and I would sometimes bring funny items like the skull to study. We don't think that Mrs. Hicks added much to my bill after Twyla and I were married. The brown turd (my Chrysler New Yorker) froze up one winter evening, as we must not have had enough antifreeze in it for the temperature. The water wouldn't circulate, so it would get hot. I was able to get it to a service station nearby and run it intermittently until the radiator thawed, and I'd then put in more antifreeze.

Twyla and I spent many hours parked on the street leading up to the nursing school's student dormitory. I always got her in on time, but some of her other boyfriends didn't.

Some of her teachers and doctors didn't like osteopaths, but five students in her nursing class married DOs. Some of Twyla's friends at the dorm thought that seven years of dating should have resulted in more action, and they encouraged her to move on. She assures me she is glad she didn't.

I started my practice in the school clinic in the summer of 1961, the same time Twyla started working at Iowa Lutheran. We took time to be married August 19, 1961, at Immanuel Church at Clarinda. John Nelson was in the wedding and caused some trouble. We gave all the males in the wedding party a set of socks and a tie. As a joke, we gave John an awful-looking tie and socks. He refused to change the items and even wore them for the wedding pictures. Neither us remembers much else about the wedding, as it was sandwiched between so many other things we had to do.

Even our honeymoon had a business purpose. We went to Denver to check out and confirm my internship, which would follow graduation one year hence. I had made no arrangements for a place to stay the first night of our marriage, so we ended up in an obnoxious motel on Dodge Street in Omaha. The second night we were in Colorado Springs and motels were tight. I finally found and reserved a room with twin beds. Twyla made me go back in and cancel that reservation, as she refused to spend her honeymoon in separate beds. Consequently, we looked until we found a satisfactory hotel.

We visited Rocky Mountain Osteopathic Hospital in Phoenix and were very pleased with the looks of that internship, and there was good housing near the hospital. We returned to Des Moines September 1 to finish my senior year, where I saw my own patients and Twyla continued to work at Iowa Lutheran.

Human anatomy was taught mostly by Dr. Marianas, a PhD. His walls were plastered with awards, some from the Queen of England. His office was glass-enclosed, super clean, and provided him a clear view of the dissection room. He left that room only to give some of us a bad time. He had shelving all about his office, above head level, which held clear, five-gallon bottles of pills. The rumor was that these were mind-altering meds and, since there were thousands, there was no accounting for any pills that disappeared. I didn't like him but got very good grades in his class. He was so lazy that he had a pattern to his multiple-choice questions to make the tests easy to correct. I would figure out the pattern and make my answers follow the pattern, even if they were wrong answers. My study partners couldn't figure out why I usually got 100 percent in anatomy tests—and I don't remember if I ever told them.

The school and Dr. Marianas must have decided to shock the freshman class each year by throwing the class into the human dissection lab on the first day. There were four to six students at each dissection table. We were told to go to the freezer and get a body for our table, and we would live with this body for the next nine months.

Ours was a large muscular black fellow who, we found out, came from the mental institution at Clarinda. Dr. Marianas was proud of the number of bodies that he had stored, and he even had enough for next year's class in the freezer. Our body would stay out on that table for the entire nine months, and it never did deteriorate. Dr. Marianas said this good preservation came from a secret liquid formulation he had us pour over the body each day before we wrapped it back up.

We were all so excited about starting this new training that the dissection lab did not bother any of us as much as one would think. Some even ate lunch in the lab and would open their sandwiches up and lay them on the body between bites. One student rigged up a pulley system to cause body parts to move when the string was pulled from a distance. The student got into considerable trouble for that stunt. We spent two to four hours each afternoon at that dissection table for the first year. I'm not sure whether students even study anatomy in this way anymore.

It seemed there were labs for everything. We spent much time looking through microscopes and studying how a muscle reacts to certain minerals. Students now would be shown computerized images and results without all that work. Learning now has to be many times more efficient, thanks to technology. My microscope was a cheap monocular that we paid about two hundred dollars for. It was fun to look through some of the other students' binocular scopes. I was amazed at how much more could be seen.

We had the option of starting our student clinic practice during the summer after our junior year, and I did. It allowed me a full nine months to build a practice, and I had a huge one. I would stay late to finish some days, which made me unpopular with the receptionists.

Everything done in the clinic was difficult and slow to accomplish. There were built-in checks and balances, but help was often slow in coming and the professors showed no sense of urgency. That was the summer of 1961, the same summer we were married.

John Nelson, Bob Ostwinkle, Ed Myles, and I would sometimes "go out" on a weekend night. I would be summoned that it was time to go by rocks bouncing off my roof, thrown by John. We caused some juvenile-like mischief during these outings for which we should have been in big trouble. One Friday night a full-sized wooden mannequin disappeared from the front of an exercise gym and ended up in one of the halls at school. On another night, several of those orange sawhorse-like blinking construction warning lights ended up on John's brother-in-law Dewey's roof. In another instance, we let loose two wild pheasants through a screen into Dewey's bedroom. I hope Dewey was a good sport. I have no idea how we ever caught the two wild pheasants or how Dewey got them out of his house. One night when Ed had not come with us, he got thoroughly soaked in his bed by a water hose through his screen.

We got into some bars where we shouldn't have been. John, quite an operator, would strike up a conversation with some of the locals. Before we knew it, we were inside. One establishment looked as though it had come straight out of the gangster movies, with the fat guy in a black suit and a hat who sat by the piano all night. On another night we were in an underground gay or cross-dressing bar watching six "beauties" dancing on top of the bar. John had to enlighten me later that they were not girls. I had too much scotch one night and missed three days of school. I got little sympathy from Twyla *or* Mrs. Hicks. I found out years later that alcohol gives me big-time migraines.

We sharpened our own needles in school and practiced giving intradermal injections to each other. Sterilization was done by boiling, as this was before disposable syringes and needles. Our sterilization must not have been good, because that same night I had an infected injection site with red streaks up my arm, most likely from strep bacteria. I went to the school hospital across the street from the clinic. It was nighttime and I was the only patient there, but I had to wait a long time. I finally raised a little Cain, as I thought I was about to die.

A young doctor appeared, who I'm sure was a senior student or an intern. He looked at my arm and then kept disappearing, probably to consult by phone with the staff physician on call. He finally gave me three shots, one of them probably penicillin. I'm glad I didn't have an anaphylactic reaction to penicillin, as treatment was very slow.

While studying one night at John Nelson's place during my sophomore year, I fell asleep on his couch. My head was on my flexed wrist and my elbow rested on the radial nerve area against the couch arm. I awakened with a radial nerve palsy, which scared me to death. I was thinking stroke or something. A clinic doctor told me that it would most likely recover with time and that there was no treatment.

I had no feeling in the thumb area of my hand and could not elevate my wrist. The wrist remained floppy, with no extension motion at all. I could not even hold a pencil. Anyway, it did start improving at about six weeks, as the doctors at school had said.

Our senior year was divided into six months of clinic, where we saw our own patients, and six months of externship (three at each of two hospitals). I took clinic first so that there could be nine months of continuous patient practice. We then went to Flint, Michigan, for three months and finally to Columbus, Ohio, for the last three months—and then graduation.

We must have been in Flint from January through March, in the dead of winter. We lived in a two-room motel-like apartment. We remember cleaning every inch of that place—it was our first home. Twyla's nursing license had not yet been transferred, so she got a good job as a waitress at a truck-stop diner. When the license finally came, she worked in pediatrics at Flint Osteopathic Hospital—but she kept the waitress job since she made more at that than she did as a nurse.

I was paid a little as an extern, and no matter how small the amount, it felt good to finally produce some income from all that study. Between my income and Twyla's two jobs, we were able to pay Dad the $125 that the engagement and wedding rings had cost.

The second externship was at Doctors Hospital in Columbus, Ohio, April through June of 1962. We lived in an apartment above the orthopedic department and Twyla worked at The University of Ohio hospital in endocrinology. We drove back to Des Moines in June for graduation, and I remember how small Des Moines seemed after Columbus.

Neither Twyla nor I remember much about the graduation, except that it meant a lot to the folks. Dad, at one time, had considered renting a bus to bring family and friends from home to the graduation. I'm glad he didn't, as I doubt there were that many from home who wanted to come. We had a little graduation party at Mrs. Hicks's and another at Uncle Eddie's on the way to Clarinda. We needed to be in Denver July 1 to start my internship. We drove from Clarinda to Denver (through Greeley) in the brown Chrysler New Yorker, with all our belongings below window level.

Chapter Five

Internship

July 1, 1962–June 30, 1963

Denver seemed like a magical place, and we couldn't believe we were actually going to live there for a year. Rocky Mountain Hospital was one of the best and most beautiful osteopathic hospitals. University of Colorado Hospital and Medical Center sat two blocks to the west, and I was in awe of the huge buildings and tax-supported medical education those interns and residents had available to them. Construction of the Spears Chiropractic Hospital had been started several blocks to the east and consisted of a number of large buildings, but it was never finished or opened, as far as I know. Spears published many pamphlets showing cures of incurable conditions with happy patients' pictures. Our doctors said they knew some of those smiling people were already dead.

Our training was called a "rotating internship," which meant that one rotated through all departments or specialties in order to get broad training. At that time, it was acceptable and even customary to start general practice after one year of intern training. There were no residencies in family practice at that time—nor were there residencies in emergency medicine yet. In retrospect, I know that internship was not adequate practical training to go into practice, and that is why the specialty of family practice was begun in the 1970s.

As interns, we did lots of history and physicals (H&P). Some powers-that-be had proclaimed that all admissions must have an H&P within twenty-four hours of admission and before all surgeries. The intent was for the patients' own doctors to do the H&P so they would be familiar with their own patients. In most hospitals, this task was quickly relegated to interns with the idea that the patient's doctor would then read the document—which often did not happen. It is difficult to legislate good medical care.

The general practice docs were happy to let the interns handle their births, so our experience in obstetrics was quite good. Since this was a rotating internship, we rotated through the departments and were responsible for emergencies when the patient's own doctor was not in the building—and sometimes even when he was.

Twyla and I were fortunate to rent a nice second-story apartment one block down the street from the front of Rocky Mountain Osteopathic Hospital. Our living room picture window faced east, overlooking a great swimming pool for the apartments on the other side of that street. We spent some time gazing out that window at all the young people having a magical time at that pool. We weren't even jealous, as it was enough fun for us just to be near such an ideal living condition. We didn't have much time to swim anyway, but we dreamed of a lifestyle like the one we witnessed across the street.

Twyla was able to work as medical nurse at Rocky Mountain Hospital. I was given a stipend in the three-hundred-dollar range, so we were able to survive and live better than we ever imagined. We loved visiting the apartments of other interns and residents so we could see how well they seemed to be living. We had never seen a dishwasher before and could only dream of owning one someday. And to have a swimming pool to use freely was beyond our imagination. We ate out sparingly and had most of our meals at the hospital or at the apartment. We found a favorite restaurant in the mountains, and having a five-dollar steak there was splurging for us. We took Mabel, Twyla's mother, for the steak and it seemed she did not appreciate the meal at all, as she thought that the cost was exorbitant.

Mabel came to visit us by herself, as Mervil may have still been in the Tuberculosis Hospital in Ottumwa. Mervil had been diagnosed with TB the week after our wedding and was in the hospital for almost two years. He appeared to be cured eventually after having a surgical lung lobe resection, and he had no recurrence. One of their cattle did test positive for TB.

I'm sure that my folks visited, but don't remember what we did. Our apartment contained only one bedroom, so we must have given them our bedroom and we slept in the living room, an act we would have repeated with all visitors. Denver was a very clean city in 1973 but appeared dingy when we visited it several years later. When we drove Mom up Lookout Mountain to visit Buffalo Bill's grave, she was quite frightened. The winding road contained switchbacks with no guardrails. We would usually visit the Coors brewery on the same outing. The last stop on the tours was the tap where beer sampling was provided to those who toured.

The doctors at Rocky Mountain were all private practitioners, with nice, high-class practices. Since the hospital had no public support, all patients were able to pay—or had good insurance. The interns were given considerable responsibility, but we still did not see much trauma or see the severe conditions that the poor or lower class would bring. The emergency room was locked, and the head nurse would have to open the room if it was to be used. It was truly a single room, and I remember being in it only a few times during the year of internship. As a reminder, this was still during the time when doctors were more responsive to their own patients and provided much more patient care in their offices. It would be almost ten years until the start of emergency medicine as a specialty.

The intercom code for a code arrest was 33, and that number still raises my blood pressure when I hear it. When this number and a room number were called, all available interns would rush to that room to perform a code blue on the patient trying to die. CPR (cardiopulmonary resuscitation) was quite new then. We had only one lecture on CPR in school, and that was by an outside guest lecturer. There were chest compressions, but air exchange was done either by mouth-to-mouth or by an E&J machine (to force air into the lungs by mask), and that machine was usually not available. Nowadays we would intubate and breathe with a much simpler bag/valve mask that was operated manually.

On one of our first days as interns, an obese thirty-four-year-old lady coded. We rushed to the bed to do the code and we all took turns at mouth-to-mouth resuscitation. The patient was vomiting, and we had to keep wiping away the vomitus in order to continue doing the mouth-to-mouth. The patient did not survive, and all of the interns attended her autopsy. When we saw the huge tuberculosis cavity at the autopsy, we were all on the verge of vomiting ourselves. None of the five of us contracted TB, as far as I know.

Another code was on a lady in her forties who was post thyroidectomy that day. She had bled under the incision, which had obstructed her breathing and circulation. Dr. Clarke (one of the interns) had scrubbed on her surgery that morning, so he recognized the neck swelling. He immediately ripped open the incision, which had been closed with clamps. This patient, also, did not survive.

In another incident, a patient of Dr. Peterson's had died in her room. I pronounced the patient dead, and we had not yet notified Dr. Peterson, but I met him in the elevator as I left the floor. I was so flustered, I guess at not yet notifying him, that I blurted out, "Mrs. Peterson just died." He knew which patient I meant and was kind enough to laugh about the mistake.

There was one internist/cardiologist who had a huge practice and was said to be making over a hundred thousand per year, a lot of money back then. The interns did not respect him as a doctor and believed that his success came mostly from his personality. He had a way of acting very concerned about the patient, but too busy to spend much time. On at least one occasion, we saw him "listen to the patient's heart" with his stethoscope about his neck but not in his ears. He gave an all-knowing grunt and told the patient that everything sounded good. This same doctor got into trouble with the government some years later and, I believe, spent some time in prison.

Twyla and I experienced our only earthquake while descending in the elevator from the third floor after one of her work shifts. That was said to be from the Rocky Mountain Arsenal inserting some toxic material deep into the ground. When that activity was stopped, so did the quakes.

The other five interns all had interesting traits and histories:

- Dick Clarke was a very good doctor, and he and his wife Treva were good friends to us. He had been in my ITS Fraternity at COMS and was in my study group of seven. Dick died of a seminoma within a year of finishing the internship.

- Ron Hansen also went to COMS with me. Ron was very quiet and not real socially active. Just before one of our classes, Dr. Elmets had asked several of our classmates who Ron Hansen was, and neither knew him. He then started his lecture to the class by asking Ron to stand and introduce himself. There were only about sixty-five in the whole class. Later, Ron did general practice in Windsor, CO, near where we would practice.

- Dr. Herrick was in his fifties. He had been a pharmacist and put his three sons through medical or osteopathic schools before he started osteopathic school himself.

- Dr. Cox was a tall, good looking, sociable son of a chiropractor. We heard that he suffered severe burns in an accident soon after internship and I don't know if he was able to continue practice.

- Dr. Jones marched to his own drummer and we could never figure him out. He was somewhat obese with long greasy black hair and was a very good piano player. He even looked somewhat like Liberace.

Both Twyla and I worked long hours during the internship year, but we did take time to enjoy our apartment. It was the newest structure either of us had ever lived in. Most everyone we knew came to visit that year. We liked The Buckhorn Restaurant and I believe that one is still in operation. Most of our guests were taken down Colfax to Buffalo Bill's Grave on Lookout Mountain as well as visiting the Coors Brewery in Golden.

We had been thinking all year about where we would practice come July 1 of 1963. We had plenty of offers to join general practices, but all were associations with no salary. The internist with the big practice did have us over for a dinner at their home, but he offered only a three-hundred-dollar-per-month salary—which was less than I was making as an intern. We began to feel that Denver was too big for us, so we looked at Hugo, Colorado, and Castle Rock, among others. The small towns were all quite isolated and remote from hospitals that I could use. Part of the draw of the small, remote town practices was that I would be forced to do the things that I thought a real doctor should do—not just taking care of rich, clean, insured people.

As the year of internship drew to a close in June of 1963, everyone knew where they would be setting up practice, except us. It was not our nature to delay planning that next step. We knew that we liked the town of Greeley, Colorado, but knew nothing about practicing there. We had heard of opportunities on the western slope. So, on the last day of internship, Dr. Origlio (a surgeon from Rocky Mountain Hospital whom I respected greatly) performed surgery on me and removed my own external thrombotic hemorrhoid in that emergency room. We got into the brown Chrysler to see Rifle and Grand Junction, Colorado. I visited with doctors at Grand Junction and was totally unimpressed. That hemorrhoid hurt a lot more than I thought it would, so that part of the trip was miserable anyway, and we did not find that magical place to practice. I think that, in the back of my mind, I had dreamed of practicing in our home town of Clarinda,

Iowa. Therefore, we headed the Chrysler east, directly toward Clarinda.

Once there, I made an appointment with the two surgeons in town. We sat in their office (just east, across from Clarinda Municipal Hospital) where I was told that, because I was a DO, they could not associate professionally with me and would not do my surgeries. I then visited our family doctor, who also informed me that if we came to Clarinda he could associate with us socially, but not professionally. It is tough enough to practice in one's hometown, but this made it look very impractical, so Clarinda was finally off the table.

We had driven through Greeley on our honeymoon eighteen months earlier, and we liked the town with the wide streets. Dr. Sprague had visited our senior class and given a great pitch for practicing in Greeley. The town had an osteopathic hospital and about ten practicing DOs there. Greeley seemed to be our best choice, so at the end of July of 1963 we headed west again in the old brown Chrysler, with the intent of establishing a practice in or near Greeley. All of our earthly belongings were in that car and were still below window level.

Chapter Six

General Practice Years

1963–1973

We should have felt uncertain, frightened, and quite unsuccessful on our drive back to Colorado in August of 1963, but we don't remember any of those feelings. We couldn't have had much money, and we knew that Twyla could work as an RN. Twyla says she started work at Memorial Hospital on the day we arrived in Greeley, but I don't remember driving her that hard.

It would be several months before I could start practice, but there is much about that time I don't remember. We had no home or acquaintances, so we must have lived in motels, but I don't know where. Dr. Sprague had a busy general practice in Johnstown, Colorado, about ten miles west of La Salle. He wanted to be gone for several weeks, so he allowed us to cover his practice and live in his house not long after we arrived. That gave us a place to stay and chance to learn a little about how a practice would be run. I could find no practices in the Greeley area that I could join—or would even want to join. We searched in Greeley and in the small towns nearby. I guess what we were looking for was to start a solo practice in a home setting or even a home-office combination, like our doctors did in Iowa. We'd had zero training in the business of starting a practice and thus, we tried to duplicate what little we had observed.

Dr. Hansen and his wife were from the area, so he had started his practice in Windsor, Colorado, by then. I guess that our rural upbringing caused us to shy away from Greeley, and we chose La

Salle, which was about four miles south of Greeley and straddled US 85. This town's population was less than a thousand but had a good number of small farms about. A well-established MD, Dr. Ordelheide, as well as a small pharmacy, were already there. It was quite a railroad town, as passenger trains still stopped in La Salle. A lot of sugar beet farming and processing took place and a pickle processing factory was nearby. One could also find several bars, several gas stations, a hardware store, a lumber yard, a small grocery store, a post office, and various other small shops and repair businesses.

My first order of business was to talk with the MD in town, Dr. Ordelheide. I set up a time and sat down with him in his office. He was much more receptive than my hometown doctors had been just one week before. He promised to send patients to me and indicated that I would see his patients when he was out of town or unavailable. He had a busy practice and appeared to be well respected. He communicated well with me throughout the years when there was something I should know about a patient. He sponsored me to the Lion's Club in La Salle, of which he was a member.

I next spoke with Mr. Norman, the owner of the pharmacy in town. He was, of course, glad to have another doctor in town, and we had a good relationship while we were in La Salle.

We badly needed a house and office to either buy or rent. We didn't consider renting, but I don't know why. We looked aggressively for real estate, but not a lot comes up for sale in a town with only two hundred houses. We came close to placing a bid on a regular house in a residential area, planning to make the front porch and living room into an office and to live in the rest. It probably would not have passed zoning, but I'm sure we didn't have any idea that there could be a problem at that time.

There was an older duplex a half block off the highway next to the lumberyard. We kept driving by that duplex and thought it would make a perfect home/office combination. The only problem was that the property was not for sale. Twyla and I went to the door anyway and asked if they had ever considered selling. Liz and Forrest Straight had not, and we thought that would be the end of that. They contacted us the next day, however, and offered the building for sale for nineteen thousand dollars. Since we had no experience in real estate negotiations, I don't know how it happened, but they lowered the price immediately to twelve thousand and we bought. They seemed very excited about our plans for the building, and perhaps did not want to sell to the lumberyard. We had no assets, so Dad had to cosign for us to complete the purchase.

The duplex was on First Avenue, the main—and only—street leading downtown. It was lined by businesses. To the left, or west, was the La Salle lumberyard. We were separated from that by only a one-lane alley which passed to the west of us and all the way north to Second Avenue where there was a nice bar. Directly to the north sat a large blacksmith shop, and to the east was another bar. Across First Avenue was another bar–restaurant combination that catered to the Mexican workers in the area.

The duplex had twin entrances on cement platforms, with three steps leading up. There were similar exits to the back. The lot was perhaps a quarter of an acre, mostly grass, with room for a garden. A large detached garage occupied the back of the lot with its entrance from the alley. A nice tall hedge separated us from the alley all along the west side of the yard.

Each side of the duplex was identical. Each had a bathroom, storage and a kitchen along the back, a large living room all along the outside, and two fair-sized bedrooms toward the middle. It had no central heating or air conditioning. Heating was by gas, with a total of six individual in-wall units, two in the bathrooms and four in the walls between the living room and bedrooms. These units had to be as old as the house. I don't know why we didn't burn that place down, with six double-burners in the walls. The wood floors were directly beneath the fires, with sparks continually falling to the floor. I thought I was pretty smart to line the floor beneath each with tinfoil, for safety.

There were always flameouts and the need to relight the gas. We just did not realize how dangerous that system was, considering that we now have professional checks of our new heating systems twice per year. There were no smoke or gas detectors in the home at that time, and they may not have been available in the 1960s.

It took several months after we occupied the house before we were ready to open the practice. We lived in the east unit of the duplex and concentrated first on preparing that for living. We remember going one block "downtown" to furnish the kitchen and bedroom from a second-hand store. We bought a used bed, a mattress, a stove, and a refrigerator, all for less than three hundred dollars. I would hate to know the history of that mattress now. I rewired the electric stove with coat hangers, and it served us as long as we needed it there in La Salle. I hope that I knew to insulate the wires in some way. It scares us to realize the things we didn't know then.

We furnished the dining/living room with a card table and used suitcases for chairs. We bought a new sixty-dollar sofa bed from the Evans Furniture Company. The sofas were made in Evans, a town between La Salle and Greeley. The sofa cost forty-five dollars without arms or sixty dollars with. I say that is still the best couch we have ever had, but Twyla did not like it. Many guests had to sleep on it. That sixty dollars may have been part of the three-hundred-dollar total we spent on furnishings. We lived in La Salle until about 1970. All of our girls were born while we lived in that duplex. We know this because we have Super 8mm movies of Pat and Pam crawling on the red carpet in their bedroom. We bought that red carpet at Sears and laid it ourselves. I'm sure we had no stretching tools except our own legs and feet, but we don't remember any problems with the carpet, and I'll bet it is still there.

As we prepared to open the office in the west half of the duplex, we decided the office was to occupy the living room and kitchen areas, but the living room needed to be divided into a front waiting room with treatment areas behind. For this project, my folks visited with Mr. and Mrs. Ralph Wagoner for a week. Ralph was a carpenter by profession, so they came to help divide that room for us. They purchased the needed supplies at the Weld County Lumber Yard, about twenty steps to the west of our office-to-be. A light wood paneling was put up, dividing the front half from the back half of that former living room. A pocket sliding door provided access between the two rooms that this change produced. I'm quite sure we had no soundproofing done between that waiting room and the treatment room. Dad and Ralph were quite happy that there were bars on three sides of our home/office, and they did visit and "got the lay of the land." I told them to never go to the Mexican bar across the street, but they went one time anyway. They returned shortly, frightened and giggling nervously. Then they told *me* never to go there. The bar to the east of us was more upscale. It had a pig roast and/or turkey fries once every month, and Dad and Ralph had a chance to experience that. Their visit meant a lot, both to us and to getting our office open. They fixed and repaired a lot of things. These were magical but fearful times.

The sign for the office was a simple black steel post with an arm holding a black metal plate, about one-foot square, that said Carl W. Otte, D.O., with "Physician and Surgeon" in smaller letters below. That sign is displayed in our garage now, just above the door to the house. We had it made by Dale's Blacksmith Shop directly behind our home. The Dale families became good long-term patients of mine. We visited with the Dales in La Salle in 2009 and learned that they have expanded their welding shop and now own our prior duplex. We made short stops at the homes of a handful of our prior patients. They treated us as if Jesus Christ had come back, and it was a real ego trip.

The office waiting room was a 12' x 12' room. The receptionist, Twyla, would sit at a small, simple wooden desk near the sliding door to the treatment room. This waiting room and the treatment room each had a door to their east, leading to the empty spare bedrooms on that side of the duplex. Those two bedrooms also had a door between them, and people could wind their way easily to the residence side. I'm sure that neither of these doors could be locked, but we never had any trouble with people wandering. After Twyla left to go to work at Memorial Hospital as a nurse around 2:30 p.m., the waiting room would have no receptionist. The early days were not busy, so I could easily handle receptionist and phone duties too. I even installed a simple buzzer that would sound when the office screen door would open. This would allow me to go to the residence side or even do some work in the backyard some days when I was open.

The treatment room was the same size as the waiting room and was suitable for only one patient or family at a time. It had a plain treatment table and a built-in white cabinet or hutch to hold instruments and injectables.

The former kitchen had great white cabinets and worked well as a lab, gynecology exam room, and supply and medication area. There was a door out the back and an adequate bathroom.

Each side of the duplex had two bedrooms. As kids arrived, we first filled the second bedroom on our side. When the third and fourth arrived, Pat and Pam, we needed to utilize one of the "spare" bedrooms in the west side of the building. Kim was moved into the front bedroom just west of ours and directly through the wall west of our headboard. We may have some pictures of Kim's first room, but it was probably quite Spartan. We likely bought another used bed and mattress and moved it in. The room would have had wooden floors, old wallpaper, and a single central ceiling light. It would have shared the gas wall heater that was in the common wall with the office waiting room. The bedroom was separated from the waiting room by a single door. The second bedroom on that side of the duplex was never utilized, except when the Wagoner family visited.

Valerie was still in a crib when Pat and Pam arrived home, so we kept her crib in the red-carpet room and got another single crib for the twins to share in that same room. Things stayed that way for a few months until we went in one morning and found Pat sucking on Pam's toe. We then moved Valerie into the bed with Kim and used Valerie's crib to separate Pat and Pam into their own cribs.

The Bruce and Jean Wagoner family visit was one of the highlights of the La Salle years. The Wagoners arrived in two cars. Dennis was stationed at Lowry AFB in Denver at that time, so some of us immediately drove to Denver to bring Dennis to La Salle. We somehow had beds and rooms for all fourteen of the family. I suppose I visited that used furniture place again. The Wagoner children seemed happy to have their own beds and not have to sleep crossways on the beds, as they must have done at home. I don't remember where we put them to sleep but would surmise that some of them had to sleep in the office area on the exam table and gynecological exam table. I'm sure that we had fun thinking all that through.

Margaret Glasgow was teaching in Greeley at that time, and she spent time at our place during the Wagoner's three-day visit. I know that I have some movies of that visit and hope to resurrect them soon and place them on DVD. We do remember that Twyla scrambled forty eggs and fried four pounds of bacon on one of those mornings—on our fifteen-dollar stove. We all attended church at Gloria Christi on Sunday morning, and the Wagoner family sang for the church. We took at least two cars and went over Trail Ridge Road on one of those days. This scenic but scary road is a part of Rocky Mountain National Park and is an unpaved road closed most of the year due to snowpack. We also would have visited Monfort's Feed Lot north of Greeley. At that time, we would still have been able to drive our cars into the lot and through the alleys that the trucks used to apply feed into the feeding troughs. None of our visitors missed this tour. Monfort's was, at that time, the largest feedlot in the world, with one hundred thousand head of cattle on feed. We would also have driven out south and east of town to view some of the large self-propelled circular irrigation systems which were new then, but common now. I'm not sure that we did this with the Wagoners, but most visitors experienced the Farm Fare Restaurant two miles north of Greeley and within smell distance of the Monfort lots. I loved their chicken fried steak and wine sundaes.

The office opened for business sometime in September of 1963. A local worker came to the door about 8:00 a.m. on that first day with a small laceration. I was *so* excited, as this would be my first patient ever and my first real income. I opened the office side door and welcomed him. The first words spoken by my very first patient at the door were, "Is your father in?" I explained to him that *I* was the doctor, and he let me suture the cut anyway. Our schooling did not prepare us for running a business or how to charge, so I charged much like the doctors had in Clarinda. A dollar per stitch. The total came to three dollars. He had insurance, so the bill for three dollars was sent off, probably that same day, to Blue Cross and Blue Shield. The "Blues" company must have had a hearty laugh when they received that bill—as it had to be the smallest ever received. They must have had another laugh when I wrote them about two weeks later, asking where my money was.

One of the early patients in the La Salle office was a local farmer who was there for some minor complaint. As he was about to leave, he mentioned that he had sustained a rattlesnake bite on his right leg that morning. Now, I had never seen and had certainly never treated a rattlesnake bite. I must have turned all shades of pale as he pulled up his pant leg to show me the bite. Fortunately, the man had a wooden right leg and there *were* two fang marks in the wood of that leg. Now the man was not a jokester, so I believe he was just telling the story sincerely as a sidebar to his visit. He had no idea how much distress his little comment had caused me. I had no antivenin and no idea where to find any. Few doctor's offices would stock it, except for those in real snake country. I administered it only once in private practice, giving the treatment to one of my pregnant patients at the Weld County ER. I realize now, after the residency and working at St. Luke's ER Poison Control Center, how little I knew about snake bites—and many other things.

It was November of 1963 when a Lincoln Lab detail man made a sales visit and told me of the shooting of President Kennedy. That made quite an impact. I'm sure that most people know exactly what they were doing when they heard this news. The same is true for the start of the Gulf War and 9-11.

Because we were not very busy that first year, we were thankful for what we had. There were days when I saw no one. Expenses were not so great anyway, and we were used to living on almost nothing. My office girl, Twyla, could go back and forth between the waiting room and the home. One of those days when Twyla had left at 2:30 p.m. to work at the hospital, I was alone and had a patient who was traveling through on his way to Denver. He said that he was an addict and just needed some IV morphine to get him back to his supply in Denver. He requested a huge dose, much more than I was comfortable giving IV. He settled for ¼ grain IV, paid his bill, and went on his way. I kept morphine and Demerol in my bag, and it had to be hard for him to watch me pull his relatively small dose out of the vial and put the nearly full bottle back. Why he didn't just knock me in the head and take the bottles, I'll never know. Also, why didn't he come back later to get my bag? I was so naïve about the nature of lower life.

I used a square black doctor's bag with many compartments—like a fishing tackle box. I was very proud of that bag and spent considerable time stocking and restocking it. The bag made lots of house calls, and it went everywhere I did. I even had some sterile trauma packs made up, having the audacity to think I would know how to use them at that time. We did have a portable oxygen tank and mask in the car, but I think it was used only once, and we have only recently gotten rid of it. I will keep the bag, and the kids will have to dispose of it after I am gone. We had intubation tubes and other emergency supplies in the office, and I felt better having them, but I doubt I would have been very effective with them at that time.

Our office used a simple pegboard system for financial records, which I had learned from Dr. Sprague. With a single writing, using overlaying papers, the receipt and appointment slip were both produced, as well as the daily ledger and billing record. We tried twice to computerize the billing, but it was just too early in the '60s and early '70s.

We had never experienced people purposely not paying their bills, and we fully expected all accounts receivable to be paid. My accordion business in Clarinda had no accounts receivable and, in fact, had no bookkeeping system at all, as people always paid fully at the time of service. We did not understand why there was money on the books now, so during the first year of practice, I would go to the homes to collect, assuming that there had been some misunderstanding. It took a while to realize that some of my new patients never intended to pay anything and would stretch the relationship as long as we would tolerate and then move on to another doctor. Many of those who were so effusive with praise and welcoming attitudes would turn out to be the deadbeats.

One memorable case stands out of a prostitute who owed five dollars for the huge shot of penicillin for her gonorrhea. I called on her at her home a number of times and received only promises of payment. Looking back now, that could have been bad for the reputation of a new doctor in town, but we were honestly thinking only of collecting the money owed or making things right if there was an issue. Her penicillin shot was another story. The more concentrated product was not available at that time. The dose was to be 2.4 million units, which was 4 cc in each buttock. We wouldn't give that much now, for fear of the buttocks sloughing. I distinctly remember her saying, after receiving that huge shot, "Do you think this will help my cold?"

Despite the above, our practice was generally comprised of the upper working class. Because of having to use the private Osteopathic Memorial Hospital, I could not take patients unless they could afford hospitalization or had health insurance. As osteopaths, we could not use the county hospital until about 1970, so we had to support our own hospital and protect the institution from deadbeats. We would not keep an OB patient unless they made a down payment of $125 to the hospital—and that usually covered the hospital bill. The charge for my delivery was also $125, but that was payable over time. Doing deliveries was a great practice builder and gave us a base of young families who remained loyal patients. We had a young practice of relatively affluent, good looking, vibrant patients. We also developed a loyal following of legal Mexican workers at Monfort Inc., a meatpacking company. These people lived in La Salle and other nearby small towns. I loved making house calls in those towns and seeing how people lived.

The medical politics in the early 1960s when I started practice was such that DOs (osteopaths) were not allowed to practice in any hospitals except their own. Most of the hospitals in the nation were run by and for MDs, who kept the osteopaths out. If one wanted to provide complete medical care for their patients, a hospital would be necessary. For that reason, upon completion of internship, our choice of practice location was quite limited. For example, I can remember only about seven osteopathic hospitals in Colorado. Greeley did have the large county hospital, which was not open to us then, and Osteopathic Memorial Hospital—which was essentially a house converted into a hospital. There was a surgical room and a delivery room on the second floor, along with about ten patient rooms. The osteopaths who admitted patients there contributed one dollar per patient per day of hospitalization to the hospital. The hospital board consisted of all the doctors who used it. When time came to make an addition to the hospital around 1967, we (the hospital board) assessed ourselves five thousand dollars per doctor—plus, we each ran a fund-raising campaign, which I hated. I don't know how much of the doctors' five-thousand-dollar pledges were ever collected, but I know we paid ours. One of the young doctors who had been there several years before us decided to leave for a residency and thus avoid paying his assessment. The older doctors didn't need the hospital so much, but I can only assume they paid their part.

One would think a small profession that was discriminated against would pull together for the common good, but that was not the case. We fought like a bunch of church members, oftentimes over nothing. There is a saying that where there are three DOs, there will be two hospitals. The approximately twenty-bed addition was completed, however, and we were proud to have it for our patients.

I am getting ahead of myself. Returning to the La Salle duplex times, the waiting room was "cooled" by an evaporative cooler in the west window. I don't remember how we got water to it. The cooler had to be loud and uncomfortable, but there were never many people waiting. Twyla sat at our twenty-dollar wooden desk in the waiting room next to the sliding door into the treatment room. She ran the phone, appointment book, and financial records until two-thirty in the afternoon on her work days. She tried to schedule appointments for the times she would be there, but we could not control walk-ins. Twyla frequently worked weekends at the hospital so she could be in the office more.

I was called over to the Mexican bar across the street one night after a fight. The injury was a lacerated cornea (front of the eye) from a chain or knife. Another night, we were coming home and carrying our four sleeping kids in the front door when we heard a man running away from one of the bouncers at the Mexican bar. He ran toward us and we heard the click of a revolver hammer being cocked. The bouncer shouted, "Stop, or I'll shoot your ass." Fortunately for us and the bar patron, he decided to stop and go back to the bar. These happenings may have contributed to our later decision to move the office and home to Greeley.

On another night we were coming home and going in the front door when Kim, age one or two, looked to the sky and said, "Cute moon."

I enjoyed making house calls so much that I may have charged less for them than I would have in the office. It was fun to have coffee with the patients and see how they lived. One of the large farmers in the area had severe angina despite receiving maximal treatment for that time. It often occurred at night, so I went often to their place in the middle of the night to relieve his pain. He always responded to a little IV Demerol and more nitroglycerine. He eventually died from his disease at about age 60, but angiograms were not yet available, nor were stents and bypass surgery.

We had, at the duplex, about five thousand square feet of grass to cut and a garden plot. We did not plant the garden after the first year, as time would not allow. I bought a rotating electric mower for thirty-five dollars from Mr. Emery at the local hardware store, and that machine with its small battery mowed that lawn for years on just one recharge each time. We didn't have much money, and the Emerys and other business people in town were very good to us. Little did we know that Mr. Emery's son Jeff would later go to the osteopathic school in Des Moines and become my partner.

We had quite a bit of company at La Salle in those first few years. Uncle John and Aunt Olga arrived in La Salle by train, and the train station was only a few blocks from our home. Our duplex was only about a half block from the tracks. The only activity that I remember with Uncle John's was a ride to Cheyenne—just to experience the nothingness of the ride. I made my old Plymouth "buck" a few times on the way to Cheyenne, which elicited quite a startle response from Aunt Olga.

My grandparents, Charlie and Minnie, came to La Salle at least once with the folks. We had a very nice five-foot hedge that separated our backyard from the alley and lumberyard. Twyla had taken to trimming that hedge and was quite proud of it, as it was dark green and thick. Grandpa offered to trim that hedge one day while Twyla was at work and I thought that would be okay. He trimmed that hedge down to nubbins and it was ugly. Twyla cried a lot when she came home that night, but I don't know if Grandpa ever knew what grief he had caused. After a long time, it grew out again.

The children were all born while we lived at the duplex in La Salle. We bought an 8mm movie camera in 1969 after the twins were born, so we do have some precious movies after that time. I have copied these to hard drives now so they can be preserved.

Dr. Patterson, an experienced family practitioner from Ault, Colorado, delivered all four of our children in that small house hospital. Twyla was an ideal OB patient. She continued to work on all her delivery days and had relatively rapid and easy deliveries. On each occasion, by the time we knew she was in labor, she was "complete" and ready for delivery. Twyla was back to work within seven-to-ten days after the deliveries of both Kim and Valerie. The delivery of the twins, Pat and Pam, was a little different. We did not know that Twyla was pregnant with twins until after Pam was delivered. Dr. Patterson then drawled, "Well, well, are you ready for the second one?" Pat was delivered breech nine minutes later. She was smaller, at four pounds twelve ounces, and Pam had already made the way, so Pat delivered easily, for a breech. Pam weighed five pounds seven ounces. Both appeared healthy and cried immediately. The placenta was like one seen with identical twins, but the girls have never confirmed their identical status with DNA tests. With the shock of it all, true to form, my first words were "That's what we get for doing it twice in one night." On a sad note, my Grandmother Otte died that same day.

Twyla had a rocky post-delivery course with the twins. The small hospital had two new incubators, so they were moved into the room with Twyla. In the days after delivery, Twyla urinated large amounts, and at about twenty-four hours post-delivery, she became confused and frightened. We thought it was inappropriate antidiuretic hormone (ADH) then, but in retrospect, I think it may have been some toxemia of pregnancy. She remained very thin for some time after the birth.

Jeff Emery, by this time, had nearly finished osteopathic school in Des Moines and was serving a three-month clerkship with me as part of his senior year. He was there for the delivery and provided the extra hand we needed that night. He had planned to fly me to Clarinda for Grandmother's funeral, but I belonged with Twyla, so we did not go at that time. Jeff and I did fly to Iowa two weeks later when Grandpa Otte died.

After about two years in the west side of the duplex, the office was moved to Hillside Center in South Greeley, about four miles away. When starting in La Salle, I'm sure we thought we would spend my entire practice life there. But the practice grew enough that the very limited facilities in the duplex were no longer comfortable. I could see only one patient at a time, and soundproofing was nonexistent. We had two more bedrooms on that side of the duplex that could have been remodeled and used. This could have served for a while, but I believe that our tastes had drifted toward something nicer, though, which would have been difficult and impractical in the old building. I don't have much memory of our thought processes at that time, so I am having to surmise. We were a little too accessible with the home/office combo, and it was becoming difficult to control the hours. I don't believe we ever considered that people would drop in after hours. We had not done that to our Clarinda doctors.

The Hillside office was nice, and we were proud of it. We rented the empty space (about a thousand square feet) and finished the interior as we desired. We divided the space into three treatment rooms—plus lab, reception area, office, and waiting room. We had professional help with the design and the furniture and were especially proud of the Torginol floor, which was a poured product and is probably still there. The aluminum sign on the front of the building matched that of Dr. Kirk, the owner, and cost $125. I believe we still have it somewhere. I had my own office and a nice desk with a hanging lamp over the desk. The furniture was all very tasteful and colorful. We were always willing to spend money for a nice office, after that first one, even though it was above our means. The cabinets in the treatment rooms were custom built at about eight hundred dollars each. They had built-in stainless-steel sinks and enclosed waste baskets, which were accessible through a hole in the top of the cabinet. The height was such that I could stand and write comfortably.

We seemed to do a lot of suturing, and Twyla continued to sterilize our suture packs with the large old pressure cooker. I didn't use gloves at that time but would do a true five-minute hand scrub before each suturing case.

We had a vibrant eighty-three-year-old man married to a forty-something wife. I asked him one time to bring a stool sample on his next visit. Two weeks later, he brought in a half-gallon ice cream container with the see-through clear plastic lid, hand-packed with his entire stool since the previous visit. We couldn't eat ice cream again for weeks. I later delivered his wife of a healthy baby, which I'm quite sure was his.

Another time, I asked a young person to "make water" in the bathroom. He brought out the container with very clear liquid which *was* water. I soon learned to be more specific and not so polite in my language.

My practice was called "general practice" in the 1960s, and I truly thought that I should and could do everything short of major surgery. I did all minor lacerations, castings, tonsillectomies and adenoidectomies (T&As), vasectomies, and deliveries. As time went on, I dropped the last three items. Vasectomies ended after a patient named their baby after me. They remained good, solid patients, however, and I soon learned that the pregnancy was not the fault of the failure of my vasectomy. There had been this party, and—well, a pregnancy resulted. They did not want to raise that love child, which was not the husband's, and abortions were still hard to come by safely. The University of Colorado could get by with more than we could, so I sent them there for a consult. They found reason to remove the uterus along with the early pregnancy.

Tonsillectomies and adenoidectomies are dangerous enough that only the most specialized physicians should do them. At one time, there were more deaths from T&As than any other surgical procedure. The doctor is working in a very bloody field only inches from the patient's airway. I decided that I could spend my time in the office doing safer and less stressful things. It was decided about that time that the surgery was neither needed nor indicated as much as previously thought.

I continued to do deliveries until the last year or two of the Greeley practice. Much joy, but also much stress, accompanied pregnancies and deliveries. When I realized that there were eight OB/GYN specialists in town doing only that, I wondered what the sense was for me to continue. How would I be able to defend a bad outcome? And more importantly, how would I live with it?

I had the time to utilize hypnosis with my OB patients and could practice it with them at each prenatal visit. Most of them still received standard anesthetics, but most would be good at relaxation techniques. One lady in particular had experienced a thirty-hour labor with her first child and was quite frightened now with the second. She had reason to be good at the hypnosis and worked well with it. She had that second baby in bed with essentially no labor.

I didn't like being aroused out of a warm bed at night to go in to do a delivery. The shivering during the drive on the way in must have been a combination of being both cold and scared. We didn't have the monitoring or the specialized help that the OB doctors have now, so I often stayed very close during the labors. The next day in the office would be difficult, but not as disruptive as it would be if I'd had a delivery during office hours. It was a relief to stop doing deliveries when that time came, which was after about eight years.

About this time, we were trying to build on to the hospital. The old "house hospital" was very inadequate for the type of practices we wanted to do, so a replacement or addition was necessary. Being a small group and highly discriminated against, one would expect that we would rally together against all the demons. The hospital had no tax and little public support, so all finances had to come from the doctors and their patients. The division was essentially The Lee Clinic against everyone else. E.J. Lee was the father and Miles Lee was the son and our only surgeon. I viewed them all to be aggressive, forward-looking, and successful. They could be quite abrasive at times and not always polite. I found myself agreeing with them more often than not, because I wanted us to be progressive and have a facility that we could be proud of. The Lees had a beautiful clinic right beside the new hospital wing with more room than the two of them needed.

When my rent lease was up at Hillside in about 1968, I moved into the Lee clinic. We dictated all our notes and had a tremendous intercom system. We dispensed medication and had our own x-ray and early outpatient facilities. There was a unique light panel beside each treatment room which told what was going on in that room. It was fun to practice in a new facility with all the new equipment as well as immediate surgical consults available to us. I did not adapt well to their complicated system and felt that help was too long in coming at times. They did allow me to bring in Nellie Roderick, an assistant who would care mostly for me and my patients.

My patients did not like the complicated clinic atmosphere. They missed the personal attention they had become accustomed to from Twyla and me. My practice fell off and I found that the Lees did not treat their friends any better than their enemies. They still ran things the way they wanted and could outvote me when needed. The final straw was when they tried to pass retirement payments to E.J. as an ongoing expense to the clinic. Jeff Emery was within several months of joining me at the clinic at that time, so I needed to make a decision for both of us. I talked to Jeff's parents and to Jeff that same night and decided to leave the clinic and take Jeff with me. I informed the Lees and gave them enough notice. Over the next several months, I noticed that some huge payments were made out of clinic income for capital equipment. My take-home pay for the last month was only six hundred dollars. Since I was buying into the clinic, the arrangements were complicated, and their lawyers did the paperwork. I bought in at one price and out at another lower price. We figure that we lost about twenty thousand dollars by being at the clinic for two years.

Osteopathic Memorial Hospital constantly struggled. Because of infighting, the true support was not always there. Fortunately, Weld County Hospital was ready, in about 1970, to begin accepting DOs on their staff. Dr. Patterson was well known in the community and respected. He was the first to apply and was accepted by a slight majority vote. I was the second to apply and was accepted. By the time Jeff came, he was accepted with no dissenting vote. I maintained myself on both staffs until I knew that all was well at County.

Jeff and I rented a small office (about a thousand square feet) on west Tenth Street in Greeley. My patients returned in droves once I moved out of the clinic. We were open six days a week, both as busy as we wanted, and even more so.

Jeff had married Nancy on his graduation day. Twyla and I got to go to the wedding, which was held in Des Moines after Jeff's graduation. Jeff was a good partner, and we still keep in touch.

Both wives, Nancy and Twyla, worked full time in the office, and we hired three more girls to help. Nellie had come with me from the clinic to the new office and was always a great help. We hired one woman who did nothing but transcribe dictation from our small Norelco machines. We dictated all office notes and all outside work and charges. This was in the 1970s when most office notes were still handwritten. Our business plan was simple, and I don't know if it was even written. We each paid expenses based upon the percentage of business we had generated that month. We operated out of that Tenth Street office for the next three years, until I left for the emergency medicine residency. We were both on Weld County Hospital staff and that worked out very well. We stayed on Memorial Hospital staff until we knew that we would both be well accepted at the county hospital.

Jeff wanted to do OB, so he took over mine and I delivered for him when he was not available. We had three exam rooms plus one small office, so it was a little tight when we were both there. We alternated as much as possible, and one of us was in the office every Saturday. I don't believe any other offices were open on Saturdays. We had no EKG, so those in need of one were sent to the hospital. Radiology was sent to the radiologist's private office. We did minimal lab in the office, but we did draw blood and collect samples to take to a local lab. We did some large lab profiles and sent those by mail to outside labs. Jeff was much better than I at business, so he negotiated the yearly lease with Leon, the landlord.

We were very busy and always seemed to run a little behind. The waiting room was small but pleasant. The business office/receptionist area was separated only by a desk and counter and a small section of wall. We used small Norelco handheld dictators with tiny cassette tapes in them to record all our patient notes. One of the girls in front typed dictation, and Twyla or Nancy would help her get caught up at times. We even dictated hospital dismissal notes and charges.

Wednesday was my day off, and it would be dedicated to assisting at elective surgeries, nursing home calls, and house calls, not relaxation.

Jeff's day out of the office was Thursdays, and this was when he would do his surgical assisting and UNC student health clinic.

We did have some fun at times and tried to make the work pleasant. I once had a very evil-sounding laugh machine. I placed it above the ceiling tile in the bathroom and would set it off when the right person was using the facilities. We did it to Nellie first, and she thought it so funny that she used it on some select patients. A person could not do that now.

We did have a burglary once in which someone broke into the rear door and stole all the cash and checks. We kept these items in a drawer in the desk, and I'm not sure if we even kept the drawer locked. We suspect that it was an inside job. We went to the bank only once per week, and the burglary occurred the night before the bank trip. It was quite a job canceling all the checks. The checks and bag were found the next spring when someone righted their boat nearby. The cash, of course, was not there.

Our receptionist took a job at the Kodak plant in Windsor. I believe that she gave us adequate notice, but on her last day, she worked until noon and just didn't come back for the afternoon. I tried to call her to see why or what happened, but her husband was very rude and would not let me talk to her. They must have been trying to make a statement, but I have never found out what it was. I had never experienced this much attitude, and in retrospect, I should have let Jeff handle that situation. The receptionist had previously worked for Dr. Sprague, and perhaps I should have investigated why she was not with him anymore.

We had to terminate another employee because she was found to be taking injectable meds home and using them on her family. She had been terminated from The Lee Clinic for similar activity in the past.

Jeff and I were always available to our own patients, except when we were out of town, which was not very often. We lived with our Norelco dictators in our hands, so we would have recorded notes about all phone calls or patient contact away from the office. The hospital had six interns each year, but we saw our own patients. There were no beepers or cell phones then, so the hospital operators were our answering service. We would tell them when we left home and where we would be, and we would check in upon arriving home again. I'm surprised the hospital would do this for us for free.

We attended Gloria Christi Lutheran Church regularly during our ten years in Greeley, and we had many good patients from that congregation. I did not do well at separating the practice of medicine from social affairs, and I found it difficult to say no to someone who was attending the same service we were. One Sunday I made three house calls "on the way home," as the patients would say. Because of this, we began to drive two cars to church, and I would leave during the last hymn so as to avoid the requests to make house calls.

I was approaching ten years in general practice. My weight was 146, and I just couldn't gain because of the hard work. Looking back at pictures from then, I looked like I was either starving or anorexic. The butch haircut didn't help any. I vividly remember the few times we did leave town and how sick I felt upon the return trip. The amount of work waiting for me upon my return would be overwhelming. There were years in which we didn't leave at all, and if we did, it would have been only for seven to ten days. The Lee Clinic, and later Jeff, would cover patient needs, but our practices were set up so that we felt much individual responsibility for what happened. The sick feeling recurred every time we approached Greeley for about twenty years after being out of the practice. It took that long to get over the anxiety that went with hearing a phone ring anywhere, especially in a restaurant.

Several years before our arrival in Greeley in 1963, there had been a major school bus/train accident a few miles east of the town of Evans. This happened at a country crossing, marked only by the wooden "X" railroad crossing signs. Twenty children were killed and sixteen injured. All who made it to the county hospital lived. Several not in the hospital or morgue at the armory had walked to a farmhouse and caused some real anxiety for their parents for a while when these children could not be found. As a direct result of this accident, national laws were passed requiring certain vehicles to come to a complete stop before crossing a railroad track. I did have one patient in my practice who had been injured in the accident and had some internal organs removed because of that day. The twenty-three-year-old bus driver was taken to the sheriff's office immediately, for his own protection. He was found not guilty, but he and his wife and child left Greeley, never to return.

I was on the second floor of the old house/hospital one evening when Dr. Sprague came up and asked if I wanted to look out the window and see an accident. Sure enough, a car had run into a parked car just under our window. It then backed up and rammed the car again and again. Apparently, there had been a domestic dispute in a home nearby and the husband decided that the appropriate response would be to totally destroy his wife's car. I must say that for a while, I wondered if Dr. Sprague had some supernatural powers where he could see the future. Incidentally, that second-story corner room in the house/hospital was where I did all of my deliveries and where all four of our kids were born. One doesn't need extensive facilities for babies to come. They have been born for thousands of years, often in much less plush surroundings—even in a manger, I am told.

After much infighting and donating, a nice-looking fifteen-bed addition was added to the east side of the old hospital. On dedication day, Twyla was dressed in her best RN uniform and assigned to show visitors around the new facility. I am sure she was very cute. She gave her spiel to one man she didn't recognize, and afterward she found out that he was the designer and builder of the new addition. He was profusely complimentary of her tour and said he hadn't realized just how good the addition was.

E.J. Lee and his son Miles Lee had historically been quite abrasive to the MD community as well as the other DOs in town. The son was residency-trained, and actually, I believe, a very good surgeon. He never developed much of a surgical referral base because of the family's personalities. I respected them, though, for their aggressiveness and desire to have things first class. I believe that Miles was eventually admitted to practice at the county hospital but am not sure if he had full surgical privileges. Two of his sons had the MD degree and have been on the Weld County staff. All of the osteopathic physicians I worked with in Greeley except one are deceased now, as far as I know. Nellie, my faithful office assistant, is also gone. She helped us originally with some childcare and housekeeping and later as office assistant at the Lee Clinic and then our last office on Tenth Street in Greeley. She would be the last of all those we worked with in that ten-year period, 1963-1973, so we have no one left in Greeley that we would want to go see, except some old patients.

For obvious reasons, I won't identify the doctors in these next two stories. If there is a lesson here, it may be that you don't know people—even if you think you do. The first doctor was in my class at osteopathic school, so we thought we knew him and his wife quite well. We were godparents to their son. He established a practice in a town about fifteen miles from Greeley at about the same time that we did ours. He had a secretary and an RN and maybe other help. One morning, sometime in 1964 or 1965, everyone was at the office except the doctor and his secretary. Patients had been scheduled and all at the office appeared normal—except for the absence of these two individuals. The wife and the RN had to notify the patients that the doctor had left town—and they had to close the office permanently. It came out later that the doctor and his secretary were amorous and had gone to Michigan where he took an anesthesiology residency and settled into that specialty practice there in Michigan. His wife and son stayed in Colorado for a while, but eventually moved to Michigan—I supposed so the son could be closer to his dad. Our osteopathic class of 1961 had a fifty-year reunion in Des Moines in 2011. I had a chance to talk with some of the classmates who knew this doctor very well. He had practices with them and had given anesthesia for their patients for the past thirty years. They knew nothing of his former Colorado life and practice or of his wife and son. The doctor and his secretary apparently had a daughter, born in Michigan. The daughter was tragically killed in an auto accident at age sixteen when she drove off a bridge. This doctor was a heavy smoker and died from lung cancer recently, back in Colorado. His wife and family were good patients of ours during the time they stayed in Colorado.

The second story involves a doctor and his wife who started his practice several years before us in a small town in the Greeley area.

He had a personality that drew people to him, and he ran a good successful business. He had built his own office just the way he wanted it in the downtown area of his small town, and he always drove a sports car, either Thunderbirds or Porsches. He and his wife had four children and were always very good to us. We were often their guests and thought that we knew them both quite well. I covered his practice when he was out of town and appreciated the business early on. He kept wanting me to join his practice, but his personality was so strong that I would have always been playing second fiddle. The way we practiced medicine was also very different. His wife worked in their office and they ran a well-oiled machine. Soon after we left Greeley, his wife took up with the local plumber who looked like Yul Brynner, and she continued to live with that plumber in the same small town. The doctor soon discovered that his wife, who did the bookkeeping, had been siphoning money from the practice and storing it away—so this was not a spontaneous event. He could identify at least thirty thousand dollars that had disappeared. I had seen this plumber through the years as a patient, and I could get no work out of any of the five female office help that we had while he would be there, including my wife.

More mystery in this practice may have precipitated the above story. This doctor took off each Wednesday, and I would cover his practice. On each of those Wednesdays, he would go to Denver for the day. This happened during the entire ten years we were in the area. He never discussed what he did so often in Denver and never invited me along. So, maybe the doctor was not such an innocent victim and "might have had it coming," as they say in the play *Chicago*. Plus, the four children all went with the wife and, to varying degrees, were estranged from their father—so maybe they knew something. We will never know, and there is no one left to ask. The doctor lost about forty pounds and took the surprise very hard. He was also a smoker and suffered a stroke sometime after and had to limit his practice.

Both of the above doctors and their first wives are dead now, and I know that one of the seconds is gone also. We never again saw the first doctor after he left Colorado, but we did stay in touch with the second doctor and his second wife until their demise.

I am constantly amazed at how friends who were so important to us at times can be completely out of our lives later. Dr. John Nelson was in my class and study group and a good enough friend at the time to be in our wedding. We had not seen him since graduation in 1961 until we stopped to see them on a trip several years ago in the state of Washington. Dr. Robert Ostwinkle was in my osteopathic class and study group and practiced in the Phoenix area. We saw him only once when we stopped at his home after he moved near Luke AFB around 1977. Another classmate, who lives and practiced here in Phoenix, we have not seen in the fifty-six years since graduation. We all get our own lives going, and what is current is so much more important than the past. I'm not saying that is wrong, it's just surprising that what seems so important at the time can go away forever. Good-bye, see you, and keep in touch don't really hold true. Truthfully, it wouldn't be practical or fun to try to keep in touch with all old friends. We would drive ourselves nuts.

In early 1973, I realized that I needed and wanted to do something different. I was so bored and tired of the self-imposed hard work of practice. I felt that if I was more trained, I might enjoy the work and have less guilt, so I even entertained going to medical school or a family practice residency. I found that I liked seeing my patients in the emergency room and was interested in what went on there. I saw some publication that mentioned a six-to-twelve-week short course in emergency medicine at Kansas City General Hospital. I contacted Dr. McNabney there and found that they no longer offered the short courses but would be starting their first ER residency in July of 1973. There were a few other ER residencies across the country, but they were so new that there were not yet any graduates of the programs. I told one of our DO interns, Gary Landers, about the residency, and he was interested in applying. The more I thought about it, the more it seemed the answer for me. I soon applied too, and fortunately, both

Gary and I were accepted for the class that started July 1, 1973. Emergency medicine was not a recognized specialty and came with no guarantee that it ever would be. We would be leaving a very large, successful general practice.

I had been to Kansas City once for the interview. After acceptance into the program, Twyla and I flew there for four days and bought a house on Melody Lane in Parkville. I had stopped seeing patients in my general practice in Greeley about mid-June of 1973 and had estimated ten days to close the practice, transfer records, and prepare for the movers. I had notified the patients by letter earlier and in person as they came in during my last few months.

The practice did not drop off as I had expected toward the end, as many patients tried to get everything done before I left. I also spent much time in conversation about transfer of records and who should assume their future care. Dr. Emery, my associate, continued the same practice but had a full caseload himself and could not possibly take all of my patients. I did much personal communication with other doctors in town, and Twyla and I hand carried many of the records to physician's offices. At any rate, the first nine of those allotted ten days were spent closing the practice, leaving just twenty-four hours to pack the house before the movers arrived. Since Twyla was my combination office manager/insurance-billing person and back-up transcriptionist, she was totally tied up with the closing of the office along with me. Neither of us were able to give any thought to the home or move until that tenth day.

We packed twenty-four hours straight and just made it but were totally fatigued when the truck left for Kansas City. After the movers packed up and left, we went to The Farm Fare, our favorite restaurant, for a steak dinner, but we were too tired and worried to enjoy the night.

We slept in the empty house that night and drove both of the loaded cars to Kansas City the next day. Twyla and I had flown to Kansas City sometime during the months before and purchased a house in Parkville, Missouri. I drove to work from there and we lived in Parkville for the next two years.

Chapter Seven

Residency

1973-1975

INTRODUCTION

Kansas City General (now Truman Medical Center) was the city hospital and unofficial trauma center for Kansas City, Missouri, in 1973. The hospital started their emergency medicine residency program that year, making it only the eleventh such program in the nation or the world. The first ER residency had been started two years earlier in Cincinnati, but at this time there were no graduates of such programs—thus no academically trained ER physicians to train us. We were trained by physicians from each of the other recognized specialties as the need arose.

There was no official recognition of emergency medicine as a specialty and no guarantee that there ever would be, by anyone. Without any official political medicine sponsors, this was a bastard residency. I had determined, however, that I would be doing emergency medicine, and I was not about to do it without more training—recognized or not.

I had graduated from The College of Osteopathic Medicine and Surgery in Des Moines, Iowa, in 1962, followed by one year of rotating internship in Denver and then ten years of general practice in the Greeley, Colorado area. By 1973, the practice had become boring, but also frightening. I found myself doing less and less and referring more. Times were changing, such that more was known and expected. I felt that more training was needed to do what I was already doing. Family practice residencies were being established, but that required three more years of training. Emergency medicine's debut occurred at about the right time, allowing one to somewhat narrow the field of study. My thought was that doing an ER residency would enable me to be afraid of nothing in that field, ever again. That was not entirely true. A good ER doc is frightened daily by the events of his practice. And I saw new conditions right up through my last day of ER practice.

Application for the residency involved a personal interview which occurred sometime early in 1973. I combined that trip with a visit to my parents in Iowa. My father rode along to Kansas City and waited for me in the ER waiting room of Kansas City General Hospital while I interviewed. Dad never did forget that wait. To appreciate this, you have to understand that my parents were from Clarinda, a small Iowa town. They had little exposure to anything prohibited in the Ten Commandments, and the strongest words ever spoken may have been "damn" or "shucks." One must also understand that many ER patients are not good people, and my parents had been exposed to very few of these during their lives. While Dad waited, a large lady came in with kids in tow and was greeted by another woman, already seated. The greeting was, "How's Amos?" The new lady, without a single hesitation said, "Oh, he was no good—so I killed him." Dad knew from the tone of her voice and look on her face that this was no joke or idle greeting. He had never been exposed to such callous talk or such disrespect for human life. Dad then needed to use the bathroom. He had just sat down with pants about the ankles when a Kansas City drunk entered the next stall. The drunk needed a place to vomit but was not very accurate with the aim of his vile-smelling stomach contents. The splatter went wide and included Dad's pants, shoes, and legs.

Dad then left the waiting room and happened upon Randy, one of the ER orderlies. Randy was a very likable person and graciously took my father on a tour of the ER. One of Randy's duties was to transport the dead from the ER to the morgue. KC General was on Hospital Hill, and there was considerable difference in elevation among the various buildings of the complex. The morgue's building sat at a much lower elevation than the ER. During the prior week, a body was being transported to the morgue when the cart got away from an orderly. The cart was upset, and the corpse was dumped into the intersection in the street, which upset administration no end. Randy proudly demonstrated a system that he had developed in which the cart was bumped against the buildings at prescribed intervals in order to avoid the previous happening. Dad enjoyed Randy's tour and demonstration immensely and spoke of it for some time. It was a new experience to see death handled in such a cavalier and routine fashion.

Randy's was one of the few names that I knew during my first few days at KC General. He was very good to me and gave me that same tour on my first day. It was nice to feel that I knew someone quite well. He was a colorful person, and I remember others wondering out loud how he could afford the two Mercedes that he drove.

Another person I remember fondly from those first few days was a young black nurse named Sara. She took it upon herself to warn the new medical residents of dangers and keep them out of trouble. I was scrubbing for a procedure on the first day and, as my habit had been in Greeley, I removed my watch and wedding ring and placed them on the small shelf above the sink. Sara came over, untied my scrubs, placed these items on the ties, and retied the knot. She said that the items would not have been there when I returned after the procedure. I soon came to realize and appreciate how correct she was.

The ambulance entrance to the ER consisted of two sets of doors with a small unheated room between. There were no automatic openers, so the ambulance attendants had to hate that entrance. This design was likely meant to be a buffer from the outside temps. The local law in 1973 must have been that all deaths had to be pronounced by a physician. This room between the doors served as a place for the ambulances to leave the obviously dead until we could find time to leave the side of the living to make the official pronouncement.

Two of the ER rooms had been drunk tanks in the past, but were no longer being used as such, probably because of political or social pressures. These rooms were lightly padded but had cement floors that sloped gently to a drain in the center of each room. There was a flush system on all four sides of the rooms which would shoot out strong streams of water, thus flushing all bodily excrements to the middle drain, undoubtedly soaking all the occupants in that tank. The vet clinic that our son-in-law Nathan used had a similar system for cleaning the cages of the meanest animals.

A Kansas City police substation occupied the ER full time. It was a rather common occurrence for patients or visitors to find themselves spread-eagled against the wall while being arrested. The constant police presence was a great comfort to the staff.

Emergency Room patient populations are naturally selected to contain survivors. They find different uses for a two-by-four or a tire iron than those on the farm. I remember being duly frightened to leave the ER and drive home the first time I witnessed the use of these instruments on human bodies.

I know that Randy and many others carried guns. I eventually did also, mostly for that long drive home. My 25-caliber, however, was too weak to penetrate even a tin can; besides, my early Ten Commandments training would likely have prevented my use of the gun.

Our residency director, Dr. McNabney, was both an experienced physician and a great human being. There were four of us who started the residency program with him and three who finished. Dr. McNabney desired that we get our feet wet early. For this reason, I was placed on duty alone on our third night there. I thought it not safe for Kansas City, but he insisted. I was really not alone, as residents from other services were working, serving their one- to two-month rotations of ER duty. There were also medical students. The ER had survived up until July 1 of 1973 manned by that rotation system. They had just not had dedicated ER physicians because there was no such thing. We moved through that July third evening with a steady diet of trash and trauma. I was seriously frightened around ten p.m. when the secretary informed me that an ambulance was on the way in with our Randy, suffering from gunshot wounds. I waited anxiously in the trauma room for his arrival. Moments later, I was both saddened and relieved to hear that he had been delivered to that room between the two entrance doors (the pronouncement area). Randy had five entrance wounds to his back and was indeed dead. If he had been salvageable, I'm not sure that I would have known what to do or could have even done it. I might have felt guilty forever for not being able to save him. The shooter had made sure that I did not have to make those decisions. The story given by the paramedics was that Randy and his pimping partner had a severe disagreement, resulting in his death in this manner. The pimping part of the story also explained the expensive cars Randy drove. Still, he had been one heck of an orderly and a very personable guy at his daytime job in the ER.

Medical Students and Residents

I must admit to some severe insecurities and self-worth doubts at the beginning of the program. I was an osteopath in an MD residency and was ten years out from academic medicine. The group of six medical students that rotated through the ER in July did not help those feelings. I could not believe how good they were already as med students and how inferior I felt. I later found out that they were a special experimental class of six who already had doctorates in some field related to medicine. They were all on their own special fast track and would be granted MD degrees in as little as eighteen months. This explained their superior intellect. I had just not asked the right questions about them.

Residents from the other specialties who had programs at KC General were obligated to spend a month or two in the ER as part of their training. Some welcomed the fast pace and excitement with regular (or at least known) hours, but many felt out of their element. Paid staff physicians would be working or at least would be available to us, which helped, although mostly during daytime hours.

General Residency Comments

The two years of residency were a frightful but rewarding time. I was finally working toward what I felt was an admirable goal and believed I would be much better for the training. The residency was actually a three-year program at that time, but I was given credit for the first year due to my internship ten years prior as well as the ten years of general practice. The severity and acuity of the patients was a new experience for me, as was the degree of social and financial deprivation of the patients. My only prior experience with gunshot wounds would have been when one of my nice private patients in Greeley shot himself in the foot. Luckily, the bullet passed between the large and second toes without doing any damage.

A resident's salary is usually a subsistence wage, so we needed to use some savings to live on during that time. We had four early school-aged girls by then, so Twyla was needed at home and could not work. Fortunately, moonlighting in ERs was allowed in our program, as it was believed to add to the broadening of our experience. I never had less than two jobs besides the residency. The ER shifts in the residency were known and scheduled far enough ahead that I could handle the extra work. Our church, however, initiated excommunication proceedings against me for lack of attendance. The two members of the church council attempted to make their initial visit as prescribed in the scriptures, but Twyla wouldn't awaken me for that.

Kansas City General Hospital was an extremely old group of buildings, the first having been built in 1870. The ER had, of necessity, been remodeled, but was still old and worn. Twenty-four/seven activity of that type in any building will make it show its age very soon. The location was on Hospital Hill, near Hallmark's Crown Center. Parking was all street parking, so each day started with a challenge on Hospital Hill, especially in the icy winters. Parking in a different spot each day would be a problem for me now as I have trouble locating my car, even after a short stop at Walmart.

Patients were preselected to be poor and unable to afford medical care. Other hospitals at that time could still turn these types away. With the unfunded government mandates that have been passed, that has changed, and now all ERs must see all comers. For this reason, there are not really county or city hospitals, as we knew them at that time. Their indigent population has been spread out to private hospitals. The government hospitals still get varying degrees of tax money for indigent care—a safety valve that private hospitals do not have.

KC General was not pretty but did give good care, partly because of its extensive residency programs. Many of the rooms were wards holding upward of twelve patients. By default, trauma was the hospital's specialty. There was no time on the street after a trauma to do a "wallet biopsy" to determine if the patient could afford the nearest hospital. City Hospital would not turn them away.

I was to give a presentation one day that required a skeleton for demonstration purposes. Thinking nothing of it, I retrieved a full-sized skeleton from an office upstairs. He was about as tall as I was and nicely set on wheels. I didn't realize that it might not have been appropriate to transport this item on the elevator until I saw the "saucer eyes" of a young man when the elevator door opened. He decided to wait, or he may have taken the stairs or left the area entirely. The next time I needed the skeleton, I put him on a cart and covered him with a sheet. That still didn't completely quiet the discomfort of the locals, though, when the elevator door would open.

Our home during the residency years was a nice four-level on Melody Lane in Parkville. Our four girls and Twyla still refer to that as one of their favorites of all our homes. We were on the inside of the Melody Lane circle and the homes had large backyards. There were no fences, so all of the yards together made a huge common playground. Kim reminded me on the phone recently that the dogs there ran free with no chains or fences. Kids were also allowed to be quite free then, and it seemed that we had all one hundred of them in our kitchen much of the time. We had moved the big red sandbox and horizontal ladder from Greeley and set them up in the backyard. I was able to plant huge pumpkins which vined around to the front of the house. One of our favorite pictures is of Pat and Pam looking out the front door with their arms around each other's waists.

The lower half-basement level had a bright red carpet, which I liked. I can remember a number of family gatherings that took place in both that room and the living room directly above. A very adequate work-storage room sat behind the lower level. Our large home entertainment center occupied the far end of that lower family room and that is where we learned that Nixon would resign, and later that Johnson would not accept the nomination for the presidency again. On one of my parents' visits, as my mother was leaving, she showed me a new nodule in her neck which, I knew then, meant that her breast cancer had come back and would probably take her life. The folks were still in good enough health then that we were able to visit family about once per month—either at our place or by traveling the 130 miles to Clarinda.

Parkville is where we purchased our first really good furniture. We bought it from Uncle Carl's stores in Waterloo, Iowa, and his people delivered it to us in Parkville. I'm sure it would have been out of their usual delivery area. I can remember the large floral couch with some side chairs, end tables, and the canopy bed.

That house is where Carolyn played a really good joke on me. We were serving Mogen David wine before the noon meal one Sunday. I gave Carolyn a really large glass and kept it full. It would disappear almost as fast as I could refill the glass, so I kept it coming. I had never seen Carolyn really drunk, and I thought it would be fun. It wasn't long, however, before I saw her slithering to the kitchen floor and babbling incomprehensibly. I thought I had really overdone it this time. I tried to stand her up, but she couldn't do it. She just lay across the kitchen stool. I felt much better later after she started laughing and revealed that she had been pouring the wine into another container and the whole "drunk thing" was an act.

This home is where Sugar died. She was a very hyper white poodle, which the girls loved. I figure Sugar must have loved me, because she would stand at the top of the steps and shimmy and pee each time I came home from work. We tried different methods of entering the house, but always got the same result. We finally put a piece of plastic at the top of the steps to try to accommodate her nervous habit. One fall day Sugar "got it" on the road in front of our house. A neighbor boy ran over her with his car. This was a big catastrophe for our family and likely our first experience with death. Twyla called me at work, but I couldn't come home early. I can well remember that ball of white fur in the small box in the garage. It was my job to do something with it after all had said good-bye.

I can't remember for sure, but I believe we took her to a pet crematory. Kim reminded me recently that the smell of burning leaves still reminds her of Sugar's death, as there was that smell in the air on that day.

Our girls would remember Grade School and some of their favorite teachers there. This seems to be their first remembrance of school. They would also remember the heavy woods in the area of the home and the many waterways not to be crossed during a rain. They have fond memories of friends there, including the Thompsons next door, the Kleibakers, and the Fergusons. They remember the swimming pool at the top of the hill right next to the shopping center, and the church only a few miles away. Mrs. Hicks, Carl, and Dorothy and their families were also there, and we did some visiting with them. Our favorite dining out took place at the Golden Buffet near the tracks, the Chicken House near the Plaza, and the revitalized Old Town area just north of downtown. We were so proud of the new Sohmer piano purchased at the Plaza. The Plaza was so pretty at Christmas. Hallmark's Crown Center near Hospital Hill was a favorite place to shop and eat, although we really couldn't afford it.

Children's Hospital

Kansas City General was purely an adult ER. In order to gain experience in pediatrics, we were to spend two months of our residency at the nearby Children's Hospital. The facility was somewhat newer and about one block up the hill from KCG. Pediatrics draws a younger staff, and their dedication to the children as patients comes easier. Much of the same abominable financial and social circumstances existed, but the children seemed to be innocent victims and not so much the cause of their own misery.

Three young nurses all named Pat worked at Children's Mercy's ER. They knew each other existed, but usually worked different shifts. Somehow, I innocently began referring to all of them as Pat number one, which they all liked. This little ego-boosting of the girls worked well for me until there was an ER party at which all were in attendance. As girls do, they compared notes about the doctors, and I became persona non grata for a while after that.

Children's Mercy Hospital not only gave good general care to the indigent but served as the referral site for the sickest and most difficult children in the area. We saw many children from normal families with two parents, and even those of the wealthy and well known, as would be the case for most specialty hospitals of this type. I shall never forget a fatality in a seven-year-old girl from a good family with parents who really cared and followed their doctor's instructions. She came into the ER awake and alive and died while in the ER from a chronic aspirin overdose. The child had been ill with fever for about three days and probably had a non-fatal viral illness. Aspirin was still being used on children at that time, and the parents had dosed the child religiously every four hours, as directed by their doctor. Because of the persistent temp elevation and dehydration, the aspirin accumulated and was not excreted. Chronic aspirin overdoses are known for being poorly responsive to treatment. One can only imagine the grief and guilt that those good parents must have felt.

Kansas City General

ER Happenings

Carlos, a man in his 40s, was brought to KCG ER one weekday by the Kansas City police. He had just been rescued from inside a closed fireplace at one of the downtown department stores where he had resided for about three days—as best he could remember. He was covered with soot and dehydrated but was otherwise awake and responsive. Carlos said he had been sitting on the chimney on the roof of the establishment three nights ago, taking pictures of the town lights, when he fell down the chimney. It was narrow, and his abrading against the inside broke his fall enough that he wasn't hurt, but he ended up inside the fireplace close to where Santa met the children at Christmas. Despite all the pounding and yelling, it appeared no one really believed that someone was behind that fireplace. He was eventually rescued by the police, who were unable to find any evidence of his camera. They surmised that he had intended to burglarize the place and thought he'd found a unique entry technique. He was not the brightest kid on the block. We hydrated and cleaned him up and then he went to jail where he belonged. We gave him an "A" for ingenuity. This story is especially meaningful to me. My father was near death and he asked me to relay the story to his roommate. That was the last request I remember from my father. I was reluctant to tell the story at that time and still wish I had been more enthusiastic about complying with his request.

Juan was brought to the ER by ambulance one morning with police in tow. His mother also appeared very soon and insisted that the one thousand dollars in his pockets belonged to "the orphans," and she got the money. Juan appeared to have been shot through the lower left leg by a high-powered rifle. The bullet exited in the front, leaving rather large bone fragments splayed out about the wound, giving the appearance of a salad or shrimp cocktail. The bullet had severed the arterial supply to his leg below the wound, so he was stabilized and taken to surgery where grafting was done to reestablish blood supply and save his leg. Juan was taken to the ICU on the third floor for recovery. Late that same night, whoever wanted him dead the first time returned. They climbed the fire escape stairs to the third floor and shot him again through the window. Juan was reclining in bed, so the bullet entered below his chin and took out his right eye. He still did not die, but needless to say, his whereabouts in the hospital from then on were kept secret. He was guarded constantly by two shotgun-wielding KC police.

Twyla was at the hospital the next morning for something and couldn't believe all the activity. Helicopters and heavily armed police swarmed the area. They didn't find the perpetrator, as he had surely left the scene immediately. They did, however, find a man hiding in the boiler room with a knife—with no relationship to the shooting. Juan was released after two months to return for outpatient care and to have his cast checked. He had a magnetic personality, and everyone who had any contact with him liked him—as is the case with many successful drug dealers. Juan was always shadowed by a small man who would have been his bodyguard. He said that he never felt safe in the hospital, even with all the police protection. He could not wait to get out and have his own protection again. The same day his cast came off, he robbed a bank and was killed.

President's Visit

President Nixon's visit to Kansas City caused some extra precautions to be taken at the hospital. We were selected as the receiving facility if something happened to him. The same arrangements must be made for any presidential visit. I know it was done in other ERs where I have been working while a president was in town. The Secret Service or FBI came several days ahead and did background checks on those scheduled to be on duty during the time the president was in town. A certain number of units of compatible blood type were to be available and in the building. The trauma room was required to be large enough to hold the president and the seven people who were with him at all times—including one carrying "the football," which was the briefcase holding launch codes for our defense system. Our trauma room did not seem to meet those space requirements, but there was an adjoining room which was deemed satisfactory. Fortunately, the president did not need our services during that visit. President Nixon had enough to worry about in 1974. A red phone had been installed with a direct line to the White House. One of our secretaries did not get the word on that and accidentally had a short conversation with someone at the White House.

New Treatment for Seizures

Interesting stories of ER happenings circulated rapidly through the ERs in that city. The University of Kansas ER supposedly received two patients with different complaints one night, both from the same address. The first was a middle-aged man with his penis severely macerated, as if it had been through a meat grinder. Several minutes later the second ambulance arrived, carrying a lady who was unconscious with a severe head laceration. This didn't make much sense initially, but a perfectly reasonable explanation surfaced later, after all was stabilized. The man sheepishly explained that the female had been giving him some oral-penile stimulation, had one of her seizures, and had vigorously chewed what was in her mouth. Naturally, he had a strong desire to terminate her seizure, so he grabbed a wine bottle nearby and bopped her firmly on the head with it. The action apparently worked. The seizure stopped, and he was able to call for help. If they had been taken to separate facilities, I wonder if the true story would have ever been known. An ER doctor ranks somewhere below a veterinarian in the reliability of the histories they are told. We listen, but then we have to sort out what is true—and often, none of it is. The veterinarians at least start with no history.

Orifice Medicine

Stories of sexual escapades abound and are favorites of audiences at medical meetings. Any lecturer worth his salt will have multiple stories and graphic pictures of objects removed from the orifices within his or her particular specialty. There appears to be almost nothing that can't be stuck in some orifice. I initially kept notes on the ones seen by us, but later these became commonplace. I'll not forget the young man with a wedding ring around the base of his penis and a severely painful and engorged organ beyond. I had no difficulty finding a nurse to use a ring cutter and give this embarrassed man immediate relief. We cautioned him to find some other means of maintaining an erection—this was all long before Viagra.

We would also see those who had inserted objects such as thermometers or sharpened lead pencils into their urethras for the same reason. One cannot fathom the variety of objects placed up the rectum—mostly as part of sex play. Doctors see these patients only when the object slips away up the rectum and can't be retrieved by the patient or the partner, if there was one. My surgeon brother-in-law claimed a patient threatened to sue him after he removed one of those large penis-shaped vibrators from the patient's rectum. The patient claimed that he had only wanted the batteries changed. I still think my brother-in-law had to have been pulling my leg.

A particularly memorable problem was the day a gentleman came in with a lightbulb up his rectum, threaded end first. No, it wasn't lit. Thus, the large round end was the part that could be felt and eventually seen—after insertion of a speculum. The problem was how to extract the bulb without breaking it and causing further injury. The ER elite had gathered about and were contemplating the problem. Appropriate consultants were called. Leave it to one of those darn smart medical students, however, to suggest the solution that worked. After adequate rectal anesthesia, a pair of obstetrical forceps was placed around the fat part of the bulb and it was "delivered," just like a baby. The bulb still worked, so we sent it home with the patient.

We had a steady diet of venereal disease cases. All had to be reported to the health department so that their inspectors could follow up in regard to contacts, to try to stop the spread of the diseases. Those inspectors dealt with the seediest people in the world, but they must have some real stories. Standard treatment of gonorrhea at that time was an absolutely huge shot of penicillin in the butt, and a standard question back then was, "Do you think this will help my cold?"

Cross dressers (transvestites) appear to have a tough and shortened life. I can remember several who came in severely traumatized. One was shot to death by a sailor who became very angry and disappointed with his date that particular evening. Anyone who has ever dated can easily conjure up various scenarios for the discovery process here and can empathize somewhat with the sailor. Truth is good—and the earlier the better.

Brandy

Brandy was a beautiful ER nurse, tall and thin, who worked at KCG. She wore the hat and hose of an RN proudly. Brandy had braces on her teeth, so even at age 28, she was trying to improve her body—which, I thought, didn't need much improving. Brandy had the hometown girl-next-door look of innocence and radiated a totally wholesome, Midwest, almost religious appearance. For all of the above reasons, I avoided much contact with her. I didn't want Brandy or anyone else to think that this married man was hitting on her. Our relationship was, therefore, always very professional and kept at a distance because of my impression of her being too pure to contaminate with my attention.

You can imagine, then, the global surprise and disbelief one Saturday morning when the story circulated around the hospital that Brandy had made a porn movie—and it was playing downtown. My wife and I were invited to a backyard birthday party at Duke's home that evening. Duke was one of our three ER residents, and his wife was having the party for him. My wife, Twyla, had never seen a true pornographic movie, so I thought it was the perfect chance to see that and then go to the party to meet some of the people I worked with. We got a babysitter and left several hours early so we could take in the movie on the way to the party. The movie did not disappoint us. The movie was named "Country Cousins" and was modeled after the story of Tom Sawyer. It started with a view from the top of the famous fence that needed painting. Tom was walking along one side of the fence and Brandy on the opposite side. I knew it was Brandy when I saw the braces. One had to feel somewhat sorry for the male porn stars. Those braces had to have hurt a lot. The movie then went through the interminably long porno scenes and progressed to the really disgusting. These scenes were all staged in very tasteful farm settings with the last scene performed in the haymow. The movie finally finished, leaving us feeling that we were leading a very boring and protected life. I contemplated what I should say to Brandy the next time I saw her. At one point, a large zit was very evident on the left buttock. I made a statement under my breath to Twyla that I sure didn't know *that* was there. Only later in the evening would I realize how unwise that little joke was.

We left the movie house and proceeded to the party, only a few minutes late. Duke's wife had arranged a very nice gathering and had invited all of the folks who worked in the ER, plus other acquaintances. Duke was quite social and had many friends. Rugged and good looking, he had many good female friends and, I think, had a special relationship with Brandy. I thought it big of his wife to invite so many of these. Twyla and I entered the gate at the rear of the house and our attention was immediately drawn to a female form rushing toward us with outstretched arms. To my consternation, it was Brandy, squealing, "Carl, Carl!" She then gave me a big hug. I didn't even know that she knew my name, let alone that I should deserve such a grand greeting. Liquor had something to do with the enthusiasm, but for me, the timing could not have been worse. I never did discuss the movie with Brandy and have been unsuccessful with my effort to find a copy of that film.

Postscript: Duke's wife was a very liberated spouse, so she invited Brandy because she just knew that Duke would like to have her there at his party.

Tetanus Case

We had a transient come in one day with a foot problem—that of never changing his shoes and socks. When the nurse did remove his shoes, the horrible smell permeated the ER *and* his toes stayed in his shoes. He was admitted to the ICU where he developed constant seizures and was finally diagnosed with tetanus. He remained in the ICU on a ventilator and constant Valium drip for days, but eventually recovered to whatever his normal state was. He must have been unusual amongst homeless persons, as most transients are hurt often and dragged to ERs each time, where the first thing that happens is a tetanus shot, so this man must have been an exception in that regard. There is almost never an immunization record available, and these people have no consistency of care. I would bet that his seizures were first thought to be alcohol withdrawal, but he was probably not a drinker. Drunks get hurt more often, and as such, he would have had plenty of tetanus immunizations.

Two ER Deaths

Pelvic fractures from major trauma can be fatal and were especially so in those early years. The pelvis consists of a circle of bone—large bones, but not especially strong. A major crush from the side (as in a fall from height or a T-bone auto accident) can fracture the pelvis in multiple places. These sharp pieces of bone can lacerate vessels in that area, plus, the exposed bone ends continue to bleed. Surgery may not be of much help as it cannot stop the loss of blood from the bones. Several procedures have been developed since that time which improve the chance of salvage. The orthopedic surgeons now place external fixation devices which approximate the fractures and arrest movement. Radiologists can also use catheter techniques which cause embolization of the main bleeders with beads. Open surgery is still not of much help.

A young man came to the ER with severe pelvic fractures from a crush injury. We stabilized him as best we could with fluids and blood and requested surgical consult. The surgical resident came and went several times, and we assumed he was consulting his books and mentors. To buy more time, I wrapped his pelvic area very tightly, which did seem to stabilize him. The next time the surgical resident appeared, he scoffed at the wrapping and removed it, and the man soon exsanguinated (bled out) and died. I believe that the tight wrap was a crude, early form of external fixation or MAST suit (military anti-shock trousers), which became standard of care sometime later.

Another sad case was that of a nice young man in his 30s who had been in an auto accident. He was unrestrained (in those years we didn't even ask about seat belts) and had struck the steering wheel with his chest. He was brought by ambulance but was sitting upright and cooperating for exams. He and I visited about how lucky he appeared to be, alive and without apparent injury. I ordered some tests and went to do the paperwork. A few minutes later a nurse asked if I knew that the man in bed four was dying. I thought she must have been mistaken but went to look for myself. Sure enough, the man appeared to be "bleeding out" from somewhere. Since that "somewhere" was most likely the chest and since Dr. McNabney (the chief of our residency program) was in the department, I opened his chest. Sure enough, there was a puncture wound in the heart that had allowed for the severe blood loss. We placed a Foley catheter in the heart wound and blew up the balloon to plug the hole and then attempted emergency repair in the ER. We were unsuccessful, and the man died within about fifteen minutes of the time we had our discussion about how lucky he was.

My moonlighting jobs during the two years in Kansas City were at North Kansas City ER and Liberty Hospital ER. I also worked a few shifts at the hospital of the Kansas City Osteopathic College. I could have stayed at either North KC or Liberty after completion of the residency. Those were the good years for getting into profitable groups, and had we stayed, we would have been much better off financially—but we would have missed some experiences. I visited an air force recruiting office one day toward the end of the residency. The decision about our next two years was made that day, as soon as I heard that I could be a flight surgeon and actually fly in fighters. The lieutenant colonel rank didn't hurt either, although the salary was only about a third to a half of my potential as an ER physician.

We sold that Parkville house to a 6'4" FBI agent and were to be at Brooks AFB near San Antonio, Texas, on July 12, 1975, for the beginning of our next two-year adventure in the air force. Kansas City was a good stay. It's where Twyla first learned to drive in a large town, and she has never forgotten.

Chapter Eight

Air Force Days

1975-1977

My residency was completed on June 30, 1975. I had considered several options for work after that time, including positions at the North Kansas City Hospital ER and at Liberty Hospital ER. I did not even consider returning to Greeley, which is what we thought we would do when we left. I had so many unpleasant memories of the hard work and stress associated with running a general practice that it was at least ten years before I could approach Greeley without becoming nauseated. We had many good experiences and knew some great people there who still mean a lot to us, but the practice had taken on a life of its own of a very destructive nature. Leaving allowed us to feel like we had just escaped from jail, and the freedom was intoxicating. We hadn't understood that people shouldn't have to work that hard to survive or be successful. Some of this may have been due to our work-ethic upbringing. By comparison, the residency seemed so easy that I had two moonlighting jobs during much of the time in Kansas City.

I had always been very interested in fighters and remember closely following the news of the dogfights in the Korean War. As a child, I would make airfields of fighters and bombers out of either two or three clothespins and would play war with them. My mother was finding these "airfields" in the closets long after I left home. The Air Force Academy had been an early option we'd considered, but at the age of eighteen, I didn't have the self-confidence to follow through on such a different vocational pathway. My folks wanted a doctor and were not much in favor of having a fighter pilot son.

My assignment in 1975 would be Luke Air Force Base in Arizona, just west of Glendale. I'd have an eleven-week temporary duty stint at Brooks AFB in San Antonio, TX, for officer basic military training, and the primary aerospace medicine course would begin July 15, 1975. The ER residency had been completed July 1, so we sold our home on Melody Lane and packed all six of us into the Mercury station wagon and the maroon Lincoln and drove to San Antonio in early July. The actual effective date of duty was July 12, so that gave us three days to get there.

We rented living space in some new apartments not far from Brooks AFB. As I remember, it was a two-bedroom apartment for the six of us. The rental had a very nice pool, which we used almost daily. It was the first time we had seen cockroaches so large—two or three inches—which we realize now were probably Palo Verde bugs. One crawled across the kitchen floor one evening and frightened everyone.

Our favorite activity was going to the many bases in the area and utilizing their shopping and other facilities. We also enjoyed eating at the top of a space-needle-like restaurant in San Antonio. An early negative experience we had was when I was stopped for a vehicle search when leaving one of the bases. The soldiers confiscated my pistol from the glove compartment. I didn't realize that they would be such poor sports about guns, and I had forgotten that it was in the car. They gave it back the next day, but I had to check it into the armory for the duration of my service. We visited the River Walk in downtown San Antonio and saw The Alamo. We attended St. Paul's Lutheran Church, which was our first exposure to a megachurch. I especially remember how good the organ was.

One weekend, we had planned to travel to the Padre Island area to see the ocean. A large hurricane came in, so we cancelled the trip. My folks had known about our plans, so on Saturday we called the folks and each of the six of us had a storm-like noise-making job to do during the phone call. The folks seemed convinced that we had gone to the ocean despite the storm, until we told them differently. That may have been a little mean, given their fear of storms.

Because of the detour to San Antonio, our children would be about three or four weeks late starting school at Luke. Through some prior phone arrangements, it was determined to be okay for Twyla to "homeschool" the kids while we were at Brook AFB. A rigid schedule of study was implemented, with many books read. The Brooks AFB library said later that the Otte family had doubled their book circulation during our time there, and they even remembered the name when I went back about a year later.

The Primary Aerospace Medicine Course at Brooks lasted nine weeks and covered the specific conditions associated with flight. We were taught how to do the physicals and administrative duties associated with the health aspects of flight. They also covered what we needed to know regarding our flying. They spent only a half day on military procedures and etiquette (such as how to salute and about-face) but told us that we wouldn't need to know much of that. I loved all of the training and ended up tied for second in the class of about seventy, which is better than I had ever done academically prior to this time.

The instructor talked about space flight and how they handled urination in those space suits. One of the class members asked, thoughtfully, if one could have a bowel movement inside a space suit. The instructor acted surprised at the question, and after a moment answered, "Well, you *can*."

Major Williams was a doctor from Clearwater, Florida, and a very convincing and motivated Amway representative. He described limiting his practice because he could make much more income from his Amway activities. He reported buying two white Cadillacs, attending enjoyable promotional meetings, and being allowed to deduct almost all travel expenses for he and his wife because they could claim to be doing Amway business at all times—which they did.

I believe that almost everyone who met him bought the fifteen-dollar Amway starter kit with the intention of doing business under Dr. Williams's line and then beginning their own pyramid. I doubt this worked for any of the rest of us. Solicitation was not allowed on any of the bases, but I'd bet Dr. Williams made it work for himself somehow.

The air force repeats the flight surgeon courses frequently throughout the years. Retention of doctors must be quite low, so they need to continually train more. Doctors are independent thinkers and probably don't make the best soldiers. Since we would be flying at least four hours per month, the air force feels they need to provide some basic survival training for flight surgeons, so we took part in a three-day course in a mountainous area near San Antonio. We were to hunt for food and encouraged to eat cactus fruit and rattlesnakes. None of us found any snakes until the last day. We were taking down our tent when we found a rattlesnake curled up about ten feet above our tent on a hill. We didn't eat him. One of the groups did catch an opossum. We have pictures of the possum being carried on a long stick between two "soldiers," and then he was roasted on that stick over an open fire. The meat tasted just like pork but didn't go far with seventy hungry people. The air force must have known about our lack of skills because at the end of the third day they brought out large pots of stew. Water presented a bigger problem. We had to chase the cattle out of the creek to fetch our drinking water and I hope we figured out to gather the water from the stream above the cattle. We boiled the water and added iodine tablets before drinking. I can still taste that iodine to this day, and every once in a while, that taste will come back out of nowhere.

The six from my group went on a long search for food on the second day. We walked several miles without success. We were quite near the western edge of the base and remembered a country-type store on that road just off the base. We felt pretty smart when we elected the two most hippy-looking of the group to climb the fence and buy some beer and food from that store. These two convinced the lady owner and her son that they were just passing through and needed to buy some food. The two made their purchase, heavy on beer, proud that they had fooled the old couple as to their true status. As the two walked down the road away from the store, they heard the old lady say to her son, "Some more of those flight surgeons." This same scenario has probably repeated itself about four times per year for many years. The two "hippies" eventually made it back over the base fence and we had quite a picnic. We got back late, but nobody had even missed us.

Late September 1975 once again found our entire family traveling in both cars from San Antonio toward Phoenix and Luke AFB. I remember that the '63 Lincoln had a bad muffler, and I worried the whole way about that. I don't know why we didn't stop and get it fixed. It could be that we didn't have the money available. I remember spending three hundred dollars on it at a muffler shop in Glendale soon after we arrived. This also may have been the trip where we had walkie-talkies in the cars so we could talk to each other while driving. We thought we were really high-tech, and I'm sure the trip was more dangerous because of our attempts at communication. As I remember, the radios had only about a half-mile range, so we could more easily have rolled down the windows and shouted. It is interesting to compare our efforts at communication then with the ease with which we do it now. Communication while driving is still dangerous, however.

We were all excited about the new life. We had thoroughly enjoyed the nine weeks at Brooks AFB and were looking forward to the times at Luke AFB. We had no home upon arrival in Arizona. We wanted to live on base, so we needed to go through the application process, which couldn't be started until we arrived. Our family was put up in the TLQ (temporary living quarters) until a home was available. The TLQ seemed quite adequate—but we had just come from three months in a two-bedroom apartment. The base had play equipment and great swimming facilities. During our time in TLQ we met the Carmens, and I believe that their daughter Amy went trick-or-treating with our girls. Twyla had made some rather extensive costuming for that event.

We were in TLQ for about six weeks. When appropriate homes became available, we would inspect the home. We had up to three chances to reject, and we did reject the first offer. We accepted the second offer, which was at 2903 Sioux. This house sat on the most northern street on the residential side of the base and was the street on which the base commander resided. The home was about 1,400 square feet in size and in very good shape. Huge oleanders surrounded the back yard. The house had no garage, but instead had a carport on its right side. Just behind the carport sat a nice little established rose garden. There were three bedrooms and plenty of storage. The kitchen, narrow but efficient, was to the front of the house and continued beyond the entrance door. It communicated quite openly with the living area, and that may be where we got our liking for the "great room" concept like we have now. We were proud to be on the general's street. He was about ten houses down and to the east. Most of our neighbors were fighter pilots or at least high-ranking. The tree in front yard was large enough to support a rope swing. We painted the rocks that outlined a front planter in brilliant white. I immediately tore up two small areas for garden which, to my surprise, grew vegetables in February. The house was only a few blocks from the base track, and I remember heading over there quite regularly to run. The rest of the family went along on occasion. Once a year we were required to demonstrate that we could run a nine-minute mile, so we had some incentive to stay in shape for that. I'm quite sure that some did not have a ghost of a chance of doing a mile in nine minutes, and I'm not sure how that was handled. The Otte girls spent much time playing at a nice small playground with equipment almost directly across the street from our home. Across a fence to the north was a vineyard and irrigation ditch. From this ditch once came a snake, which we diagnosed as a copperhead and which Valerie ran over with her bicycle wheel. Twyla and I were visiting with some neighbors in the street when Valerie came up to tell us about the snake. She was tugging at our clothing and trying to talk. True to our "be seen and not heard" attitude about children, we finished our conversation before she was allowed to inform us of her big find. Someone, maybe Twyla, killed the snake with a shovel. Carmen's house was on the street behind us, just thru the oleanders and several houses to the east. Amy and the Otte girls wore a regular path between our homes.

Litchfield Road divided the base into the military operations side on the west and military housing on the east. The base hospital was on the housing side on Litchfield Road at the entrance to the housing. For once, work was close enough that I could ride my bike or walk. The entire base was well patrolled by the MPs, so it was not an option to speed or break any laws. Our piano tuner came twice during those two years, and each time was stopped and questioned about his intentions. He was a seedy-looking character with a not too good-looking vehicle. He told us we'd have to get another piano tuner next year. Imagine how he would be welcomed now. In 1974, Twyla wanted our Christmas picture to be of the four girls in front of a large cactus on the operations side of the base, so she arranged for a professional photographer. They entered the west side of the base, which was okay as our cars were marked, and we could take in guests as long as we were responsible for them. He took the pictures, but when he tried to leave, the base was locked down and he was told no one would be leaving. The poor guy spent the next two hours with our girls in the car unable to leave for any reason. Once again, we would need a different photographer for next year—we probably should have asked Aunt Vera.

This account is being written with family in mind. Thus, someone may have heard my stories a few times. I'm sorry about that, but what I remember has probably been reinforced by being told. Some of the stories may have some entertainment value or family history value in the future, so I want to get them down before they are forgotten. I have decided to do this in some type of chronological order and possibly draw out the emergency medicine stories later.

We have described the military years as an ego trip, and that it was. I was allowed, in some ways, to fulfill a lifelong dream of flying fighters and actually be paid for it. The military folks were better to us than we deserved, for the most part. I entered with the rank of Lieutenant Colonel, which allowed us to bypass much of the "payment of dues" necessary to obtain that rank, but this did nothing to address my deficient military knowledge. Also, being saluted by most everyone and outranking most of those in my environment did nothing to keep me humble. However, I was reminded daily that those around me had more knowledge and experience in military fields, and that tended to keep me grounded. No one ever made me feel bad for those relative deficiencies.

In addition to the observations above, being a flight surgeon provides some additional status. Flight surgeon's offices are usually separated from the rest of the health care area and, at Luke, were at the very front of the hospital. There were usually four flight surgeons at Luke during my time there and somewhere between thirty and fifty other physicians, as well as thirty dentists. The flight surgeon is looked upon as the ultimate physician, at least as far as the air force's mission is concerned. Any problems connected with the flying mission would be addressed by that office. People ask if we do surgery because of the word "surgeon" in the name. Surgery is not a major part of what the flight surgeon would do, although they certainly do some surgical procedures if needed. I don't know the origin of the name, but "surgeon" was likely used in the name in order to ascribe more status to that specialty in the military.

At Luke, the flight surgery office occupied the front southwest portion of the hospital. This was most practical, because corpsmen and a flight surgeon were to respond with an ambulance to the flight line for each in-flight emergency. An in-flight emergency would be called any time a plane was landing with any unusual condition. Examples might be anything—illness or injury to a crewman, warning lights of malfunction in the plane, or any known damage or fire in the plane. A number of vehicles are assigned to respond, including fire and rescue personnel. The plane would usually "take the barrier," which meant the tail hook was put down and the plane would be stopped by a huge cable strung across the runway, similar to landings on an aircraft carrier. The reason for this is to stop the plane in a known location so the team could more quickly get to the plane and the pilot. These responses were usually for routine matters that required no attention, but the in-flight emergencies occurred almost daily. Eight emergencies in a single day are the most I remember responding to. Several times planes came in on fire or with other significant damage, and those times would reaffirm the need for the responses. One plane came in on fire and was immediately foamed down by the fire truck. The pilot then slipped on the foam during his egress and fell to the tarmac, fracturing his ankle. The cockpit, even on the smaller fighters, is ten to twelve feet above the ground. They climb into the cockpit via ladder or specific staggered steps on the plane.

As you can imagine, the above played heck with any office schedule we might have had. In addition, we were encouraged to fly as much as possible. If a back seat opened up during the day, our office was notified, and we would cancel out and go fly. In addition to flying, the flight surgeon's duty included annual physicals on all who flew as well as on their life-support personnel. We would also take care of their general health and injuries, in addition to their families' health. It was the only time in my thirty-eight years of practice when almost all my patients were college graduates. This made for a very rewarding but sometimes challenging practice. They wanted answers and reasons for things. I can't imagine how things must be now with the internet available to them.

Caring for flyers is and should be a specialty. The flight surgeon is to fly so that he or she can become familiar with the special effects of flying on the body. Examples of these effects include oxygen deprivation, spatial disorientation, g-force effects, fatigue, effects of medications, and barotraumas. An upper respiratory infection can be serious or fatal for a fighter pilot. If the hollow cavities in the head (e.g. sinuses or middle ear) are congested so that air cannot move freely in and out of those spaces, extreme and disabling pain can happen with altitude changes. You have probably experienced ear or sinus pain with altitude changes when you have a cold, even when changing altitude in a car or upon landing in a commercial plane. This pain would be of more rapid onset and seriously amplified in a fighter, given the rapid altitude changes. For this reason, a flyer is grounded if he has an upper respiratory infection (URI) and not put back on flying status until cleared by the flight surgeon *and* the central air command. That is one of the red tape items of the job. Central Command would sometimes overrule the local office and not allow a pilot to return to flying status based on our conversation with them. Flyers did not like being grounded because it put them behind in their classes and, if too frequent, it could affect their careers.

Luke AFB is almost purely a fighter training base and can be thought of as the pilot's last stop before combat. A pilot receives extensive training at other bases prior to their arrival here. This would involve academics, simulators, and other jets used for training. They were at Luke to learn to fly the F-4 and F-15 during the time I was there. Nearly a hundred West German pilots were on base at that time learning to fly the F-l04. Luke was the second largest fighter base in the world at that time—Russia had a larger one, but that has likely changed by now. The number of planes at Luke in the '70s was about three hundred, and I surmise that the number is about the same now. We had a reserve unit flying the CH-53 helicopters and had some smaller copters for rescue operations as well. In 2003 it was the F-16 and F-15. The old reliable workhorse of the cold war (the F-4) has been retired. Now, Luke has become the main training base for the F-35, and they are much louder than the previous fighters here.

The F-4 was a truly remarkable plane for its time. It was one of the best in the world at what it did. It could do ground attack to support the troops on the ground as well as hold its own in aerial combat. It could break the sound barrier and could be configured to deliver atomic weapons. To do this, the plane would approach the target fast and low (50-100 feet). The F-4 would then pull up (pop up) and throw the bomb forward. It would then continue pulling up along that same path until it was on its back, heading in the direction from which it had come. It would thus accomplish a 180-degree change in direction in order to most effectively get away from the blast. Fortunately, for the world, all of this practice has never been needed.

True to my nature, I became deeply engrossed in the business of the flight surgery office and caring for patients. The first month had nearly passed, and I had not yet been in a fighter plane. The hospital commander, Colonel Johnson, found out, and by that same afternoon I had a ride. The pilots typically brief for the flight for two hours prior and debrief for about an hour after each flight. We were to be a flight of four, doing ground attack practice that day. During this maneuver the planes would place themselves in an approximate square, with the target in the center of one side of that square. The F-4 approaching the target from the nearest corner would dive in to attack and then recover back to the previous altitude. Thus, there would always be a plane attacking or recovering as we all took our turns on that circling square. They briefed that we would all do four attacks from each of three angles and then finish off with four more dives, strafing with machine guns. I sat in the pre-briefing thinking they wouldn't do this to me on my first ride (sixteen dives) but they did—and it was okay. In addition, when recovering from the dive, the pilot would roll over, upside down, so we could look at the ground to see what we had hit. I was somewhat disappointed at what we saw. I had expected huge explosions, but the pilot explained that we would be using only practice bombs for this phase. People on the ground would also report verbally to us how each run had gone. That job had to suck.

Once that first flight was over, I loved every minute of it and flew much more than the required four hours per month. The most time I logged in any month was twenty hours. Because of the briefings associated with the flights, each hour of flight logged in fighters ate up considerable time. The hours that would count toward flying were only actual hours in the air—so pre- and post-flight briefings did not count. I was assigned to the 426th, which flew F-4s, and the 58th, which flew helicopters. The 58th flew frequent evening and night missions into northern Arizona, and we saw some game and some Indian ruins which may have been difficult to get to any other way. I loved shooting the machine guns out of the helicopter doors. We didn't shoot at the game, but at targets on the Goldwater Range. Most of southwestern Arizona is one big shooting range, used by a number of our bases. Because of the number of planes using the range, it is rigidly controlled, and one has to be cleared in order to use it. One would think that no one would live on the range, but it does have a sparse population. There is an auxiliary base at Gila Bend, mostly for use by any planes that could not make it back to their home base.

One exercise with the fighters consisted of trying to shoot down a drone plane with machine guns. A small drone would be attached to an F-4 and once in the air, this drone would be let out on a two-thousand-foot cable and towed. The other planes in the flight would then attack the drone and attempt to hit it with their 20mm machine guns. It was harder to hit than one would think, and sometimes the drone would win—for a while.

My favorite activity was air combat practice. You know what it is like if you have seen the movie *Top Gun*. For machine-gunning, the best position to be is at the enemy's six o'clock position (behind him). We were close on the tail of an "enemy" once when the F-4 ahead of us lost an engine—it flamed out for some reason. He slowed dramatically, and we had to pull up sharply to avoid a collision with him. That pilot used the Gila Bend airfield since he had a major problem, and it was thought safer for him to get on the ground as soon as possible. We slowed down and stayed on his wing until he landed safely. Staying on the wing seemed a little theatrical, and although it does make good movie material, there was nothing we could do to help the injured plane. It makes tremendous sense in enemy territory though, in order to discourage the enemy from trying to finish off a partially disabled plane. We did land our own F-4 at Gila Bend once, but I don't remember what type of emergency we had. A bus transported us back to Luke after a long wait, which was not much fun.

My one F-15 ride was an air combat mission. The F-15 was fairly new then and did not allow much room for non-essential flights. After a first flight the custom was to be greeted with a champagne party, and we have a picture of that from my flight.

One mission was to experience high-altitude flying. We approached fifty thousand feet, which is about the body's limit without a space suit. Oxygen is fed through the aviator mask under positive pressure, and the voices sound like Donald Duck. The "unloading," or the experiencing of weightlessness, is done at that high altitude. One is not really in weightless space yet, but one can feel the experience by allowing the plane to slowly lose altitude. I became very frightened at that time because my g-suit began filling and was becoming very tight. I squawked my concern to the pilot in that duck voice and he immediately told me to get my emergency manual off the suit-inflator button. Sure enough, in the weightlessness, the manual had drifted over onto that button, and removing the manual allowed the suit to deflate. G-suits inflate automatically when g-forces are detected, but the button in question is an override so that we could inflate the suit manually if the mechanism ever failed or we felt we needed more suit pressure. The automatic inflation always worked so well that I had almost forgotten about this button. Luckily, this pilot must have flown with some novices before on this altitude exercise.

The flight manual that shifted onto the button is a Bible-sized yellow book that all flyers have in their possession any time they fly.

It contains a summary of what should be done to respond to various in-flight emergencies. Our job was to read the section referencing the occurrence to the pilot while he tried to correct the situation. That book would be about the only thing not tied down in the cockpit.

In movies you see pilots flying with their oxygen masks slung off to the side. This doesn't happen in real life. The mask is applied tightly before leaving the ground and doesn't come off. It feeds progressively more oxygen appropriate to the altitude, and when an altitude is reached where plain oxygen is not enough, it is fed under positive pressure, much as medical oxygen is sometimes fed to oxygen-starved patients. We want our fighter pilots to be as alert as possible. Oxygen starvation does not bode well for thinking and acting. Fighters change altitude quickly; as a matter of fact, the F-15 can break the sound barrier going straight up. Hypoxia can be quite subtle, and putting on an oxygen mask is not one of the things a pilot should have to remember to do. Besides, a little hypoxia may contribute to his forgetfulness. The oxygen system appears to be quite dependable and is one of the flight systems necessary to give him (or now her) the edge.

We were flying in an F-4 one-day in the southern portion of the range. I looked down and told the pilot in alarm that we were on the Mexican side of the fence separating the United States and Mexico. The pilot made no immediate correction as I had expected he would. His comment was, "What are they going to shoot us down with?"

The cold war was still in full swing in 1975. Everything we did would be compared to Russia at that time, and there was much discussion in briefings about the Russians' planes and their capabilities. It was supposedly known then that Russia had LAFB targeted for a 25-megaton nuclear bomb, with another for the Southwestern Air Defense Command cement block house, which was also on base (and a half mile from our house). These bombs would have been twenty-five times the strength of the atomic bombs that we dropped in World War II. These would have wiped the base and all its planes and people off the map. Upon each takeoff during that time, the crew would know their divert base where that plane would be flown in case "the balloon went up" while on that flight. It would be a strange feeling to look down at our homes and families and hear the pilot say, "Well, if the war starts today, we will be going to Albuquerque"—or wherever.

I was working through a busy office schedule one day when the office was informed that a flight had come available to South Carolina and they needed a "back seater." My patients were rescheduled, and I must have gone home to get into my flight suit. I loved that suit and wore it any excuse I had. They cost about eight hundred dollars at that time. The suit had lots of zippered pockets and was fire-retardant, as were the gloves. We were to take an F-4 across the country for some repair work. As careful as I am, I'm surprised that I didn't want to know more about what was wrong with that plane. The flight was uneventful, except for two or three landings at bases to refuel. After landing at the base in South Carolina, we were debriefed and then a beautiful girl in a convertible transported us to our quarters. We ate at the officer's club that evening and stayed overnight and then were to take another repaired F-4 back to Luke the next day. We were in the plane and ready to taxi when a strange request came over the radio. The ground crew said they really wanted to know one thing before we left. They obviously had placed bets and wanted to know which one of us had slept with the girl who had picked us up. The captain had to admit that it was neither of us. We assume that this was not the first time they had placed bets amongst themselves about the situation.

The flight back to Luke proved more eventful. The F-4 lunged to the side at one time during the flight. We elected to fly on in to Luke with the plane rather than land earlier somewhere else. The conversations with ground control about our problem, of course, activated the in-flight emergency system. It was a strange feeling to look down when we did our base leg and see all those emergency vehicles on the field, realizing that they were there for us this time.

The plane landed without mishap and I never did hear what had been wrong with it.

The F-4 and the F-15 have two engines each with 15–25,000 pounds of thrust. This is the same size engines found on many of the commercial airliners. The difference is that the fighters are much smaller and lighter. Upon takeoff, or turning and recovering from a dive, the body is trying to travel in the direction that it had been going but is forced to change direction with the plane. This is called "pulling g's," or forces of gravity. At two g's the body is pushing against the plane as if it weighed twice the person's weight, etc. The pilot or navigator is taught to bear down with one's lower body muscles to counteract the g-force and its effect on circulation. While g's are experienced, the body's blood tends to pool in the legs, thus the brain might not have enough circulation to continue to function if g-forces are not counteracted. There is also a g-suit, which is put on over the flight suit. It has multiple bladders, which blow up with air under pressure when g's are experienced. The pressure from the suit is also graduated—in other words, the amount of pressure exerted by the suit is relative to the amount of g's being experienced. An experienced pilot in good shape can stay conscious up to about nine g's.

The F-4s and F-15s had afterburners to be used in situations requiring even more thrust than that provided by the usual engine activity, such as in takeoff or combat. When the throttle was pushed full forward, a rocket-like fire would be ignited behind each engine, which gave the extra thrust. Fire could then be seen coming out from behind the engines, especially visible at night. This was not an economical way to travel because it used a tremendous amount of fuel, so it was used somewhat sparingly. One also wants to have enough fuel to get back home. As I remember, the planes burned about a thousand gallons of jet fuel per hour, and could fly one to two hours, depending on the mission.

One doesn't just get into one of these planes and fly away, like in the movies. The flyers were attached to the plane in eleven places.

There were shoulder, lap, and leg straps attaching him to the ejection seat. Each lower leg was buckled to the front of the seat in two places—to prevent their flailing upon ejection. Then there was also the communication attachment for the microphone and earphones. Oxygen was plugged in for the facemask and compressed air to the g-suit. The oxygen, air, and communication all had to be friction connections (much like the pressure connectors that a farmer attaches from his tractor to equipment he is pulling) so that these would all disconnect during an ejection.

The ejection seat is a complicated but wonderful and necessary part of the modern fighter. It is meant to be utilized when the plane cannot be safely landed and the flyers must escape the plane. The sequence can be initiated by the flyer pulling either of the two rope-like rings that are located on the front of the seat or above his head. The reason for two triggers is that there may be conditions of the plane or the pulling of g-forces that might make it impossible to reach one or the other of the initiators. Once either of those rings are pulled, the canopy is blown off and the seat is blasted out and up by two rockets underneath the seat. The speed of the eject must be sufficient to get the aviator away fast enough that he is not struck by the tail of the plane. This takes a real kick in the bottom and is one aspect of flying that is not practiced but is taught extensively. The force is such that fully one in four who eject experience spinal compression fractures. In order to provide some familiarity with the system, we had to practice being ejected on an upright rail at Brooks AFB. The force was provided by a strong spring and was as close as possible to the real thing, but still fell short of the true ejection experience.

Both aviators in two-seat planes have a handle to rotate before takeoff to activate the ejection seat and to set the system so that either of them could eject both aviators. If something happened to the pilot, such as a bird strike or a wounding, the back seater could still eject both. The air force did not want flight surgeons to attempt to land a plane if the pilot was disabled. We were to take the plane out over our eject area (which was the White Tank Mountains) and eject both of us. I was always a little insulted by that plan, as I thought it would be safer to attempt the landing. The ejection sequence, in two-seat planes, was such that the rear person went out first. If the pilot went first, his seat rockets would burn the back seater. The flyer is separated from the seat soon after the ejection and then is brought to the ground by parachute. There is a backpack that stays with the pilot, providing survival equipment, flotation devices, and weapons.

The ejection seats do work as advertised and do save lives. There were a number of plane crashes during my two years at Luke, and in each case, we went out to pick up live pilots. There had been three F-104 crashes just off the end of the runway in the year before I arrived, and all ejected safely. In the years we lived in Sun City Grand, there have been six or seven F-16 crashes, and all have walked away, to my knowledge.

Ground ejection is possible, but not recommended. The explosive force beneath the seat is enough to propel the flyer upward about three hundred feet, such that the chute has time to open and give the occupant about one swing in the air before they hit the ground. The need for ejection while on the runway is not a good thing, but my pilot and I discussed that very thing one day while taxiing an F-4 after landing. We had smoke in the cockpit but decided to do a rapid ground egress instead of a ground ejection. That proved to be the right decision for that situation. It takes about nineteen seconds to get everything disconnected and get out of the plane. We did that on the spot and nothing more happened. It would have been a bad decision to do the risky ground ejection, as it turned out.

All who fly are required to demonstrate proficiency at rapid egress from the plane every three months. The time target was about nineteen seconds, but I'm not sure that I ever made it out that quickly. We also periodically had to practice water landings and show proficiency at getting out of all the hardware after being pulled backward into water.

There were very sophisticated flight simulators for the pilots to use and which we could access on an "as available" basis. These were essentially cockpits set on movable mechanisms with 360 degrees of screens surrounding the cockpits which simulated the flying environment. They were so realistic that some pilots who did not get sick in the planes did vomit in the simulators.

There were one or two flights that should have meant more to me than I understood at the time. There was an auxiliary field called Aux 1 about ten miles north of Luke Field at which we practiced instrument landings. A controller on the ground at this abandoned landing strip would monitor the practice landing, as the pilot would be purposely blinded during the instrument practice. The controller would communicate with us by radio and was there for safety as the pilot's backup eyes during this practice. There was no plan to actually land at this dirt strip, but everything was practiced except the actual touchdown. Little did I know that twenty-eight years later we would have a home in almost exactly that same area. The Aux 1 field was actually covered over by the Surprise spring training facility and the city pool and library. Aux 2 was north and west of our house.

I have heard that there were about fifty of these dirt auxiliary Luke airfields built during the World War II training that took place at Luke. There were literally thousands of planes at Luke then, and more room was needed for training than could be provided at the one base. The planes at that time could utilize the short dirt strips, but today's jets cannot. Most of the extra bases have deteriorated from neglect. We still hear occasionally of drug runners using these old strips to land their drug-smuggling planes.

The military intends to respond to humanitarian missions and uses these as part of their readiness practice. On one weekend, some illegal aliens from Mexico were lost in the desert of southern Arizona. Some of their number had died and the rest were scattered. We utilized our helicopters to fly crisscross patterns across the area and we did find survivors. This same scenario still plays out frequently on the news in Arizona, so the problem has not been solved.

Another sad mission was to investigate a civilian crash site at the top of a mountain near Payson. A plane with four on board had crashed and was inaccessible by ground and too high for the civilian copters of that time. It was midafternoon, so only a few hours of daylight remained. The crash proved to be in the scrub brush at the very peak of the highest mountain in the area. The air was so thin up there that the copter blades did not have good lift properties. We approached the scene with a large CH-3 as well as a smaller Huey helicopter, but there was only room for one of them at the site. I believe that it was the smaller Huey. The crash had been very hard, and only small pieces of the plane and small, scattered body parts remained. There had been no fire, so we wondered if there had been any fuel left, although it appeared that they had just not cleared the peak. We needed to hurry. Night was fast approaching, and by morning animals would probably have consumed the remains. We separated the body parts of the four victims, three adults and a female child, into four separate body bags as best we could. I picked up a teddy bear and placed it in the bag which we thought was the child's. I remember picking intestines off the brush and guessing into which bag it should go. A local rancher and his Collie dog appeared on the scene while we were there. So, as darkness fell, we prepared to lift off with the additional weight of four bodies, the rancher, and his dog. Everyone sat with their feet on body bags, and I remember sitting in the copilot's seat looking down through the glass bubble at the brush beneath us. We attempted to rise off, but the brush just blew in the wind and stayed in contact with the Plexiglas at my feet. We hovered several feet off the ground and could not gain altitude. The pilot finally pushed forward so that we flew off the ledge without ever gaining any altitude—and it worked. We delivered our cargo to the coroner in Payson and felt happy to be back at a lower altitude where the air was thicker and the helicopter blades had something to grab onto.

Part of the deal when I joined the air force was that I knew to which base we would be assigned. Because we would move there with an active young family in school, I wanted to see the base and the area before we came. I must have flown out by myself, arrived at night, and rented a car. I intended to take Van Buren to Grand and Grand toward the base. My sense of direction became mixed up and I went a long way east on Van Buren. I could not believe that it was wrong. After asking directions several times at the motels on Van Buren, the correct westerly direction was taken, and I stayed that night at one of the seedy motels on Grand, somewhere near Glendale Avenue. It's possible they weren't so seedy at that time. Little did I know how much of our life would be spent near Van Buren and then Grand. I was not very familiar with citrus, nor had I ever seen much of it. There was this beautiful large orange hanging right outside my second-floor motel window. I don't believe I had ever stolen anything in my life, but I convinced myself that it would be okay to sample that produce. I brought it in through the window, peeled it, and tasted the worst orange I can ever remember. It must have been one of the decorative sour oranges.

I must have seen what I needed to of the base and housing the next day. I was so impressed that the Luke school pupils could eat their lunches outdoors and use the playground most of the year. We have great pictures of these picnic tables, which we used to help the girls become excited about the move and their new school.

In talking with Kim recently, she indicated that the air force years provided her most vivid childhood memories and were her favorite years. Kim was selected as the outstanding student at Luke School while in the fifth grade. That honor usually went to the most senior sixth graders, so Kim's recognition may have put some of the sixth graders' noses out of joint. The general (base commander) himself presented the honor. Another student received an award for being at the school for six years, which must have been unusual, given the mobility of the air force families.

The good base experience caused Kim to at least consider the Air Force Academy, and we did go there later to visit before she chose her college. Thirty positions are given to students who want to be lawyers each year, but there was no way to be sure of getting into their legal program.

The girls all remember specific things from these years. The rope swing I put up in the tree in the front yard, the park across the street, and the running track at the end of the street. One of the girls remembers the rocks in the front yard that we painted white, and that we had a garden and quite a successful rose garden. Someone also remembers burying the pet fish under the tree. Pam was impressed with the stingray car driven by the general's son. She recalls decorating our bikes for the Fourth of July parade and the huge wiener roast at the track, hosted by the general. Pam has a memory of me riding my bike to work with the flight suit on. The Brownies leader made an impression on the girls because she couldn't start the meeting until her soap finished on TV. The girls found some Indian Head pennies in the oleanders behind our house.

Barb Carmen, Twyla, and all the girls except Kim went to see a dairy in operation on Olive. They brought some goat milk home and let Kim drink it at supper before they told her—and she got mad. Twyla tells of the night we got all the girls up to see a huge frog or toad outdoors. The girls collected about a hundred small toads or frogs in a paper sack and brought them in the house—to save them from the rain. One of the girls lifted the sack later and the bottom of the sack was wet and stayed on the floor. The hundred little amphibians had apparently peed in the sack and were now loose in the house.

We were all in Flagstaff at Little America Motel for a medical meeting when my mother died. We drove back to the base and I flew back to Clarinda. Twyla followed later after arranging for child care.

The flight surgery office was in charge of medical security for the base. One day, one of our technicians came up with a positive test for poison in the base drinking water. It turned out that the test was simply too sensitive, and the water was all right. It caused a lot of commotion, though, as all water was shut off. I remember an F-4 taking off at midnight carrying samples of water to another base for further testing. The whole episode takes on a new meaning and importance now after 9-11.

Flight surgeons were assigned several squadrons to be their responsibility. We were encouraged to party and mix with the pilots so we could stay in touch with their stresses, observing them unofficially for any dangers to their flying. The squadrons would hold a party for almost any excuse. The air force years are the only time I have owned a full-out black tuxedo for winter and a white one for summer wear— and they did get used. Remember that these were sharp, hand-picked people, and their parties were such good-quality fun. They were much like Leno and Letterman in their ability to turn current happenings into comical events. They would go to lots of work for a laugh, if necessary. One party especially stands out. Three of the pilots took video of themselves riding tricycles, simulating fighter pilot training. A live turkey was passed around and the lowest scoring squadron on the shooting range had to care for that bird for the following week. Twyla enjoyed the social life. The privileges of higher rank appeared to carry through to the wife also. An "in thing" that would happen at nearly every party is that someone would holler "slug bug" and all the men would fall to the ground and under tables, if possible. The last one down was to buy the next round of drinks. I was always protected and don't remember ever having to buy the round, even though I must have been left standing with the women, especially at first. There was an officer's wives club that met monthly, and Twyla was treasurer of that organization.

Many memories have surfaced by talking with Mother and our girls. Bud and Barb Carmen adopted Catherine Carmen during our two years on base. We were good friends and visited with the Carmens often. We were also friends with Fishers, Browns, and Ogrens, among others. We frequented the Officer's Club for meals, especially on Mongolian barbeque nights. We still go there with our neighbors, Bob and Shirley Cooley here in Sun City Grand, to eat. Bob was a retired air force fighter pilot with access to the base, and he could take us on.

We attended the black church on base several times because we enjoyed their music and enthusiasm so much. Our white, mostly blond family must have stuck out like a sore thumb on those Sundays. Our girls saw nothing but fighter jets for the two years on base. They take off and land at over a hundred miles per hour and disappear into the clouds in just a few moments. We could not shoot the machine guns above a certain speed because the plane would outrun the bullets and could shoot itself down. The entire family went to Sky Harbor Airport once to pick up visitors. Little Pat, who was five years old, looked up at a commercial plane as we were approaching the airport and said, "Oh look, an airplane stuck in the sky."

All four of the girls took piano lessons from the wife of a pilot who had been shot down in Vietnam. She had a chilling tape of his rescue taken from the helicopter's radio conversations with him while he awaited their arrival. The pilot was hiding in a hollow tree and in the background of his radio transmissions could be heard the voices of the North Vietnamese and their dogs as they searched for him. The rescue was successful and I'm sure there is more to the story. The husband was an instructor pilot at Luke. Most of the pilots I flew with had combat experience in Vietnam, and some wore jackets stating the number of missions they had flown over there.

At that time many were still missing in action from the Vietnam war, and MIA bracelets were big. I distinctly remember seeing a teenage girl as a patient in the flight surgery office who wore one of the bracelets. As a matter of conversation, I said to her, "Oh, I see you have one of those MIA bracelets, do you know the person on it?" I had no words to follow up with after she said, "Yes, it's my dad." This story, as well as the rescue story above, still give me chills when I think of them.

My dad and mom visited us once while we were on base. They were not too thrilled about my occupation when they observed what the jets would do. I'm sure they had never seen planes doing anything like what they observed on that runway.

Twyla was area coordinator for Girl Scout cookies and needed to go off base to pick up the order—for the whole troop. She asked Dad if he wanted to go along to pick up some cookies. Dad thought they were going to pick up a box or plate of cookies. He was so surprised when Twyla carried out case after case until the red and black van was totally filled. He said later that he would have helped if he'd known there would be so many. We have had many good laughs about this.

Another episode on that trip was when Dad and I went to the flight line with his camera to get a picture of the row of F-4s. We heard a voice over radio or intercom stating that someone was taking pictures at our location. Soon, security was all over us. I thought they would take the camera or film, but they must have decided that any spy would have a better camera than we had, and they let us keep our picture.

Paul's and Larry's families visited us on base on their way back from a driving trip to Las Vegas. They had driven the five or six hours to arrive and, true to our usual form, we put them back in our car to go eat *somewhere close*. We drove them over to Bill Johnson's Big Apple at Nineteenth Avenue and Bell, which must be about twenty miles. At that time, Bell was a simple two-way oiled road with not much between here and there. Upon arrival at the restaurant, Paul gave one of his typical low-level relaxed understatements, saying, "I'm glad we didn't go *somewhere far*."

Most doctors at Luke had to take their turn as MOD (medic of the day), which meant being responsive to the emergency room for twenty-four hours. We would spend our usual day in the office and then finish the twenty-four hours by going to work the night in the ER. Emergency Medicine was my specialty, but I believe I hated the duty as much as the rest. We were not a true Emergency Department, being more of a night clinic, but we were still subject to some horrendous cases. Admission capabilities were limited, so the bad cases would be transferred to civilian hospitals or air-evacuated to the major military centers. I never liked it when my hospital could not give total care to whatever came in. One case that stayed with me is that of a young airman who crashed his motorbike and slid on his face on the asphalt. He had ground his face down to the extent that I could put my fingers into his exposed frontal sinuses. One wonders what they could do for that and what his face must have looked like. His world changed forever for him in just an instant. He seemed unhurt otherwise, so he is probably surviving to this day somewhere.

Bob and Cheryl Fisher and family were at Luke for about one year before we arrived, and we overlapped about one year. We found that Bob's mother (Huseman) came from Yorktown, Iowa, and that he is somewhat related to both Twyla and me. We became good friends, and Bob was willing to teach me much and help us adapt to military living. Bob and Cheryl were the first to expose us to Arturo's for good Mexican food. Arturo's was located about five miles southeast of the base on Van Buren and was a favorite pilot hangout. We weren't supposed to wear our flight suits off base, but we did there, as we would often go for Mexican food directly from work. Our family went there frequently during our two years at Luke and even after our return to The Valley in 1980. Another place we enjoyed visiting was the town of Litchfield Park, about one mile south of Luke. The main street at that time went through downtown and was lined with alternating palms and citrus, a sight often seen on postcards. I remember flying down main street, very low, in a flight of four F-4s one Fourth of July. The townsfolk were used to seeing fighters, but seeing and hearing them at just above treetop level must have been memorable. A bypass takes traffic around town now to the west, and they have tried to duplicate the tree pattern on that section. The original street is still intact, going through town and past The Wigwam Resort, but is not so well traveled now.

Air War College is a study course offered by the air force and is a good thing to take for career advancement. It can be taken at the home office in Virginia or by weekly discussion meetings on base. These were attended and run by high-ranking officers. In-depth discussions of world events and the air force's view of its place in those events occurred in this course. I took the course because I thought I might be making a career in the military. We had to write two essays in order to graduate. My first was a thoughtful paper on the world energy situation and our dependence upon foreign oil. My solution to the problem recommended very high taxation upon energy use in the United States. I thought that it could, almost overnight, solve our dependence upon foreign energy, provide some great tax income, reduce driving and accidents, and give the US incentive to develop alternative sources of energy. I still think this would be right to do, even now. My paper received the highest grade and some good comments. My second paper was completed after I was out of the service and in Cedar Falls. It was not nearly so good and barely passed, but I am a graduate of Air War College.

Each air force plane accident requires the convening of an accident board, which consists of one member from each of the disciplines involved. The six-to-eight-person board always includes a flight surgeon. When we were assigned to the board, the case became our only duty until the case was closed, which could take a month or more. Bases that are short on flight surgeons could receive one assigned from another base to serve on their board. Bob Fisher was sent away to other bases twice for this duty, but I never was.

I was on one case where some tree material was lodged on the underbelly of the plane, which is considered an accident—as they are not to fly that low. That was a short case, and I'm sure it was determined to be pilot error. The fix would be to make some policy or procedure to prevent recurrence, if not already in the books. I am always amazed and amused at the efforts that the military and civilian boards will go to in order to come up with preventive measures, even if it grounds the fleet or suggests restrictions which are not consistent with the big mission.

My other board duty lasted about a month. The case was complicated, involving the loss of an F-4 somewhere above Lake Pleasant during a refueling exercise. The fighters can only operate for an hour or two upon the fuel they carry. With our worldwide commitments, refueling is becoming a most important capability. Planes are sometimes refueled just before entering enemy territory. The large tanker plane (the gas station, as the pilots like to call it) has about a twenty-foot boom that can be extended from its tail area. The boom actually has small wings near its distal end, which allows the refueling officer to fly the boom, to some degree. The fighters have an opening into the fuel storage system near the canopy—in the F-4 it is just behind the second seater. The pilot opens the cover and tries to match the speed of the tanker. He has to get close enough that the nozzle can be flown into that opening by coordination of his speed and the limited movements of the boom. When connected, they rapidly transfer large amounts of fuel and then the fighter moves out to let another in to do the same dance. Something happened one day, and the boom struck the canopy of one of our F-4s, possibly breaking it. The boom was broken off and the pilot and copilot in the F-4 ejected. The tanker was otherwise okay and went back to its base and landed. The F-4 kept on by itself until it crashed near the top of an isolated mountain north of Castle Hot Springs. I was dispatched by helicopter, along with several of our corpsmen, to retrieve the pilots. It was stressful not knowing what would be found. The flyers had a location beacon, so we knew roughly where to look. They were lucky to have landed on hillsides where they could somewhat control their landings, and they were unhurt, except for a few "cactus bites." They required nothing medical, so all we had to do was take them back to the hospital for their mandated physical exam.

The accident board on this case ran for over a month, as there was so much material to consider and so many site visits in unfriendly country. The actual crash site was in an inaccessible area, even by helicopter. A team from security hiked four hours by foot to secure the site and remove any live ammunition that was left. They set up communications and stayed at the site until we had retrieved what was needed over the following days. We then scoured the area, from the ejection site to the crash, for ejection seats and helmets. Some searching was done by helicopter, but much had to be done on foot or by vehicle. Another captain and I made a number of trips in four-wheel-drive vehicles, including his Toyota truck. This is where I developed my tremendous respect for Toyota products. The road to and past Castle Hot Springs is strewn with large boulders. One four-mile segment requires rumbling over river rock in the creek. The few people who live up in that area are friendly but remarkably isolated and noncommunicative, considering that they were only thirty or forty miles from Phoenix. The inhabitants of one cabin were very excited and friendly to see us land by helicopter in their yard because, they said, "Grandma went to the hospital in a contraption like that when she broke her hip."

We had not yet found the twenty-foot boom that we knew had come off. Several of the locals had told us it was in the back of Jed's yard, and gave us directions to his place. They were apparently not used to giving directions or talking to strangers, so we had considerable difficulty finding Jed's place. Once there, however, he was very cooperative. Sure enough, there was that huge item about fifty feet behind his cabin, lying right where it had landed. He explained that he had watched "this thing" come out of the sky and land there. He had no idea what it was, and one has to wonder what he thought and why he didn't contact some authorities—as it had been there for several weeks. It had to have been the biggest happening around there for a considerable amount of time. Jed's area had rudimentary roads, enough that we were able to get a truck in there to do our retrieval. Castle Hot Springs Road continues on north and then curves west to intersect Highway 60 (Grand Ave.) at Morristown, and that segment is more passable.

I have pleasant memories of two meals that the captain and I discovered on the above missions. One was a bar at Lake Pleasant Road and Carefree where we had the largest and best-tasting hamburger ever. I would suspect that some beer went with it. That bar is open to this day and still serves the same food. Twyla and I have eaten there several times since we moved to Sun City Grand and it is not far from us. It is named Wild Horse West and has had the same owners since my visits there in 1977. Castle Hot Springs Resort was also still open at that time (1977) but was closed for a seasonal break then. A small cadre of about six employees stayed to guard and clean the place. We somehow got invited to eat a noon meal with those folks and had some interesting discussions. Some of the resort burned several years later and it has been closed since. It was a beautiful place with palms and hot springs and had been visited by President Roosevelt at one time. ASU owned it, the last I knew. Large buildings still stand there, empty and seeming entirely out of place—almost surreal. It was protected by huge guard dogs the last time I was there and seems like a perfect place to make drugs or do anything where you want no visitors. Some of our kids and I did go up to this area one Christmas some years back. I wanted to find where the plane had been and possibly get some souvenir parts from it. We had no luck even finding the site. We also noted that recluses who did not care for company had replaced those friendly people, and they guarded their isolation with wire fences and dogs.

The two-year air force assignment was to end July 11, 1977, and we needed to make some decisions. My air force duties did not involve much emergency medicine, and most of the air force emergency rooms were really night clinics. I needed to do real emergency medicine in order to validate my residency and become board certified in the specialty. The incentives I was offered to stay in were a twenty-five-thousand-dollar signing bonus and the choice of assignments to bases in Germany or Holland. These sounded almost too good to pass up, but one must remember that the cold war was still very real then, and the fear was that Russia could roll across Europe within a few days—and we wondered whether the US could or would attempt to stop them there. I was very aware of these catastrophic possibilities since we had discussed the "what if" scenarios in briefings, and certainly even weekly in War College. In retrospect, either of these tours would have been a tremendous growing experience for the entire family, but they carried a significant risk at that time. The air force was also considering starting its own emergency medicine residency program in 1977. I was one of only a handful of residency-trained ER physicians in the country, and possibly the only one in the air force. Being assigned to start the residency program at the "Big Willie" hospital at Lackland AFB in Texas was another possibility. I was not ever interested in academic medicine and didn't believe that I deserved the responsibility or had the teaching abilities that would be needed. In looking back at this and the civilian opportunities over the next ten years, it is evident that we severely underestimated the value of my services. Being residency trained and certified in a new, rapidly growing and vital specialty meant that one could almost write one's own ticket in the business. My only goal, however, was to be the best ER physician that I could be. I did not realize the financial rewards or respect that would go to those who ran the programs or groups. Many of these leaders would be involved with the business of medicine and the politics, and that did not appeal to me. Taking advantage of some of the business opportunities in the next years (which will be discussed later) would have made for a much easier and secure life for us, however.

The last night on LAFB for Twyla and me was spent at a party in our honor at the home of Major J. D. Brown and his wife Louise, attended also by Major Ogren and his wife Kim. These men were in my 426th squadron. I had spent many hours with the men, flying and doing squadron business. As couples, we had many good social memories. J. D. and Louise pulled off an elegant and intimate dinner that lasted over four hours, with multiple courses of food and drinks. J. D. and Louise impressed us greatly with their ability to make the courses flow with seemingly little effort on their part and no outside help. We didn't remember either of them ever leaving the table. One of the drinks was served in a tall, expensive, multicolored long-stemmed Waterford glass, and that is probably why Twyla got the set of six for me now—which we look at a lot but seldom use.

Chapter Nine

Post Air Force

Cedar Falls, IA

1977-1980

After leaving the Air Force, I needed to decide where to do real emergency medicine. In preparation for that decision, we had traveled to two places during the last six months. Our choices were between Palm Springs, California, and Waterloo, Iowa. We quit telling people of our two options, as they would double over in laughter upon hearing our dilemma. No one could understand why there would be any decision to make. They assumed it would be Palm Springs. So we went to Waterloo. I would work at Schoitz Hospital ER for a group that staffed multiple ERs in Iowa. Robert Singer, MD was my employer and immediate boss, and we still stay in touch with them. The main advantages of moving to Iowa were that both of our families would be closer, and Uncle Carl and Aunt Ada actually lived in Cedar Falls. The job involved no administrative duties. I would just be an ER doctor on salary.

In retrospect, had we taken the Palm Springs fork in the road, I would have had considerably greater income and status. Another doctor and I would have been starting the ER for one of the Palm Springs hospitals, meaning I would have started down the path of greater administrative responsibilities. And because of location, we would have seen the affluent and famous. I remember that the contracts with the hospitals at that time were that we would be paid eighty-five percent *of our charges*, a deal which would change later as the makeup of ER patients changed. Our family visited Palm Springs before making the decision to not move there. We noted that the schools seemed to be filled with minorities (the politically correct term would be "very diversified"). It appeared that there were two classes of people in Palm Springs—the rich who vacationed and lived there, and the poor who provided the services for the industry. The kids would have had to go to private schools if they were to not be a minority. We stopped at a housing development and found that the homes were five hundred thousand dollars and up. We didn't know homes could go that high, and I think that was the final straw.

We had several weeks before my job started on August 1, 1977, at Waterloo, so we took a family vacation to California. We stopped at the 426th squadron on the way off the base on July 12, 1977, to pick up some pictures from J. D. Brown that he had taken at the party the night before. We then headed for California by way of Palm Springs, which was on Interstate 10, going through the Goldwater Bombing Range over which I had spent so much time in the past two years. The range covers most of southwestern Arizona, so the military has plenty of room for practice to occur while still avoiding several interstates and sparsely populated communities. We also had no way of knowing what was happening on the range that morning that would mean so much to us.

I don't know how they found us, but when we arrived at the motel that first night in San Diego, a message awaited us from Major Ogren. Major Brown and a student had been killed that morning in an F-4 accident on the range. They had been doing a low-level (fifty foot) nuclear release practice run when something happened. There is not much chance to recover from that low altitude. They ejected but did not survive. We had the next few days planned with the usual kid's activities in California, so I did not go back, and I have wished many times that I had. It would have disappointed the kids significantly to drive right back, and I did not want to leave Twyla alone with four small children in California. J.D.'s wife Louise later got a job as head of protocol for the Air Force Academy, which she held for years. We have seen her only once since, when she came to Phoenix. The Ogrens are in Tucson, and we see them occasionally.

We visited Sea World, the zoo, and Disneyland. I have little memory of the trip except that we met a man at our first motel who claimed to be the original Spiderman in the movies. I also remember the kids riding on an elephant. We then drove all the way back to Iowa in the old Mercury station wagon. We had sold the maroon Lincoln for two hundred dollars before leaving the base. Twyla and I had been back to Cedar Falls sometime earlier to purchase the house on Fourth Street. The schools were within several blocks, and we could see them from our house.

I'm sure that we had promised the kids a new dog when Sugar died in Kansas City. We had obtained a small black poodle while on base and named him Luke. How we got that dog to Cedar Falls I don't remember. I never did like that dog. He had the nervousness of a poodle and temperament of a pit bull. He would choose one family member to protect each day and would bite any one of us who approached that person. I was in the habit of kissing the girls as they slept whenever I came home from work late. I had to stop that, as Luke would be under the covers of his "protectorant" for that day and I about lost my face a few times.

Several of the houses we had looked at on our house-hunting trip to Cedar Falls would have been catastrophes. One was a large castle-like house on a big knoll with lots of grass spilling down the hill on all sides. Mowing or getting up to it in the winter would be a nightmare. It had some small nooks upstairs that I thought the children would enjoy playing in, which shows how one feature can almost sell a house. Another house had a swimming pool, and we even got to the point of bidding on this one. Neither house would have been rational choices in Northern Iowa. Denny Leahy (Pam's husband) sensed that we were having trouble picking a house and guided us to the one we ended up purchasing on Fourth Street. Twyla remembers that we had gone back earlier to find a house and secure the job. We landed at Cedar Rapids and took a small plane with a rough ride to Waterloo, where Uncle Carl picked us up at the airport. On that trip I stood on some nice grass near the schools and looked back at the house that we were considering. Some angry-sounding people were hollering "fore" at me, and I couldn't understand why. I had never played golf.

Our move to Iowa was a very busy time. I was taking board certification exams and finishing my War College paper as well as starting a new job and home. Soon after arrival we were invited to Steve and Cynthia's wedding in New Haven, Connecticut. Larry, Irma, Twyla, and I flew there and rented a car. Actually, Twyla rented the car because the rental company would not accept either Larry's or my credit cards. We rented a nice larger car, probably because that was all that was available. Uncle Carl gave us a bad time (in jest) because that was the car he wanted, and it was not available for him. We enjoyed the trip very much and have talked about it often. We stayed in a quaint, charming New England hotel. The wedding was beautiful and a new experience for us all. Irma and Twyla wore long dresses, which was the custom for the area. Cynthia skipped around at the reception throwing flower petals out of her basket. The salad was served after the main course and then sherbet "to clear the palate." Larry's family joined us to ride a train or subway to downtown New York where we saw the usual sites and ate at Mama Leone's.

Iowa had great schools as well as hospitals and churches. The elementary and junior high schools that the girls would attend were about two blocks away. We could see them out the front of our house, across a large park of green grass—well, in the summer, anyway. They had a great indoor heated pool that the Otte girls utilized to the max. Swim team was an important part of their lives there—and they all did very well at it. The snow drifts were sometimes higher than the school roofs.

The house at 1803 West Fourth Street was a great family home for the three years we were there and provided many happy memories. It was light brown with dark trim, split-level, with three small bedrooms. The utility room off the kitchen had folding doors, and that is where we would have to pen Luke when anyone came. Our green and yellow fiberglass picnic table sat on a very small cemented patio on the east side, just off the dining room. The girls remember me shoving about four inches of snow off that table so I could lay on it and suntan with aluminum foil around my face for better reflection. A good tan in the winter in Cedar Falls would be unusual, and we didn't know then how bad it was for the skin. Both the front and back lawns of the house were all grass, which required considerable mowing with our electric corded mower. Large trees occupied the front yard. I planted four or five fruit trees in the back, but we weren't there long enough to realize any fruit. I dug up a small area along the back of the lot for a garden, and we had some produce from that. This garden is where Mrs. Corning told Twyla she saw me putzing one day. That really insulted me, as I thought I was working. Her garden was *much bigger and more productive* than mine and everything they did always came out golden. I was so indignant. The Cornings were good neighbors, but it wore us out to watch all their activities. They had a plum tree that was loaded with fruit when we arrived. Those plums were *so* good, and we had as many as we wanted each year. Some of our girls helped the Cornings put on a lobster feed for a party at their house once.

Twyla and I must have stayed at Uncle Carl's when we flew there to hunt for a house. I suspect that we all stayed there for several days until our furniture arrived from the air force. Uncle Carl and Aunt Ada were a great support system for us while in Waterloo/Cedar Falls. I told them initially that this would not be a permanent move, as we were still moving frequently at that time. We were guests at their place quite often, and I remember a number of nights when I would go over alone. Uncle Carl and I would sit in those orange leather chairs, sipping a Seagram's VO-7 and talking.

Part of our reason for moving back was to be closer to family again while the kids were growing up. We had a good opportunity for that while in Kansas City and again two years later. It helped the girls to appreciate Clarinda and the Midwest lifestyle so much that they almost consider Clarinda their home also. It seems that this feeling has passed on to some of the sons-in-law as well. My mother Martha died while we were at LAFB, so we appreciated the fact that we had been close enough while in Kansas City to have family times. My father Orval was still alive for most of the Cedar Falls years, and all of Twyla's family and my sisters were within easy driving distance from Cedar Falls. Doug and Carolyn and family in Des Moines were the most accessible, so their place was invaded frequently. Their three girls were close to ours in age, which made for some good times for the seven of them.

Our house on Fourth Street was a split-level with three small bedrooms and only one full bath. Pat and Pam were put in the smallest bedroom, which wasn't much more than a hallway. We purchased bunkbeds from Mueller Furniture, as that was all that would fit. I later tried to make the room appear larger by making one of the side walls into a mirror, with one-foot pieces of mirrored glass tile. It didn't work out well, as we had trouble getting the tile to stay on the wall. I would come home from work after a midnight shift change and find the entire family in bed with Twyla. One time, I didn't take them back to their beds, but made myself a bed on their floor. The girls felt so bad that there wasn't room for Daddy in his own bed. They still remember that we would awaken them by carrying each to the bathroom every morning. We painted the outside of the house during our three years there and did it all ourselves.

The lawn was considerable work, as the entire lot was grass except for the area that the house sat on. That is the way most lots are in Iowa. The large shade trees had superficial roots growing near the surface, which made the lawn uneven and hard to mow.

We were in Cedar Falls for three of the worst winters—1977, 1978, and 1979. The snow would be so deep in the driveway that we couldn't throw it any higher. The United States Postal Service kept sending us notices that we needed to expose our mailbox so they could get to it to deliver the mail. The girls talk of how they shoveled the driveway for hours, and then the city would come along and plow the street snow off the road, having no place to put it except in the driveways. One time, we were partly done when someone came along with a grader and finished it for five dollars—he said he would have done the whole thing for the same amount. The dam of snow that the plow would leave across the driveway entrance was almost impossible to move, as it would be partly melted slush that would quickly freeze into a solid two-foot-high wall. Fortunately, we had made some contacts while in the air force near Phoenix, and I knew there would be a job, so after three years of this, I made that call.

We had sold my beloved maroon Lincoln Continental before leaving the base, so we needed a car for me to drive upon arrival in Iowa. Twyla would use the station wagon for the multiple activities of four girls. The Mazda dealer in Waterloo had a light blue metallic hatchback that had a back seat and looked good. It was brand new and in the three-thousand-dollar range, which seems impossible now. It would get good mileage but was a standard shift, which I thought would be no problem. The salesman took me for a ride in it. He drove it off the road down a steep embankment (about twenty feet deep, as I see it now) and back onto the road. He must have done that maneuver before and knew the car could handle it. The vehicle was rather low-slung with small wheels, wide apart, so it was probably quite stable. Anyway, after that demonstration, you couldn't have kept me from buying that car. I'm sure I thought I would do this to other people who rode with me, but I never did. By the way, no one else in the family learned to drive that standard shift. We practiced on empty roads in new areas of town and maybe even on that golf course, but it remained solely my car and was sold after three years when we left for Phoenix. It was a great little car.

The girls and Twyla got up early on very cold days for swim practice. They were quite active in swim team and traveled all over the state for swim meets. I was not much help with that due to my work schedule, which usually involved seventy-two hours per week, with sleep in between. Twyla walked quite regularly, sometimes in very cold weather. I went to the Unidome to run on the coldest days. The place was so big that I kept thinking I didn't belong there, but it was used extensively by the locals for exercise.

The wood appliqué on the Mercury wagon doors was peeling badly, to the point of embarrassment for all of us. I priced the reapplication of the material to the doors at the dealer and received a bid of one hundred twenty-five dollars per door. and I didn't even ask how much to replace that wood look on the entire car. Twyla got some contact paper that matched the original wood appliqué and we applied it in the appropriate areas for about thirty dollars. The wagon looked like new, and we were so proud of it then.

I forget why, but sometime later we decided we needed a new mode of transportation for the family. We all remember the day I sold the Mercury and watched it drive away. We'd owned that car since Greeley and had many good memories with it. We purchased a new 1979 red and black Dodge van. We just fell in love with that van when we saw it at the dealership in Waterloo. Maybe we weren't dressed very well, but for some reason, we could not convince that salesman that we could afford that van. We really tried to buy it, but they just blew us off. We went to Granger Motors in Granger the next day. This small dealership in an old business building was obviously just getting started. The first words we heard from Tim, the owner and only salesman, was "I'm going to sell you a car today." We thought, "Tim, you don't even know how true that is." He ordered the same van that we had seen in Greeley and paid extreme attention to every detail we wanted. We were so happy with that van and with his service. We went to Granger for all the checks and maintenance while in Iowa. I would have a list of concerns and requests on each visit, just like a neurotic patient. They must have groaned each time they saw me, but they were always professional.

The town of Granger had two water towers. One day I asked why that was. The immediate reply from behind the counter was, "One for hot water and one for cold." I think my reply was, "Oh." I'm sure they've enjoyed answering that question many times before. On one of our recent travels through Granger we stopped to talk with our old friend Tim. He now has a large new dealership out on the freeway, and we were so happy to see that he had done well, as he deserved to. Tim, however, had changed, and he either did not remember us or did not care. We have noticed that this happens with many old acquaintances when some time has passed. A friend is maybe *not* forever.

There was good eating in Cedar Falls, as there is in all of the Midwest. The Brown Bottle was—and still is—an Italian food place with good lasagna. It is very busy and fun to visit. The Broom Factory is a restaurant in an old factory and has atmosphere. It sits along the river, and we usually get seated where we can see the river and the old railroad bridge. It was owned by the family of one of the nurses I worked with at Schoitz ER, which made it even more interesting. We visit it each time we go through Cedar Falls now, and the food, especially the onion soup, is still good. We entered the restaurant several years ago and noted a huge four-by-five-foot painting leaning against the front counter. It showed a large Arizona home in the desert, and I recognized it as one that I saw off in the distance every time I drove to Wickenburg to work. The lady who owns the Broom Factory said the home was a ranch home that she and her former husband had built. She said that the house had over twenty thousand square feet under its roof. It had been sold, and she wondered what had happened to it now. I asked around and was told that an orthopedic surgeon owns it and has seventy horses on the ranch. We hope to see it sometime.

Nazareth was our church during our three years in Cedar Falls. Lutherans are big in Iowa, and this church had about three thousand members. We were not real active due to our busy schedules at the time. Pastor Larsen, the minister, was a very dynamic person. He remembered everyone's name and could keep our attention on the sermon more than anyone I have ever seen. He said that as people age, they get more like what they used to be. The sermons had current local information and shock value. He thanked the Almighty in one of his sermons for the conversion of two of the current members of the congregation, whom he named. He said that these two men used to go to Minneapolis to see who could drink the most and lay the most women in one night, but now they are married and "going straight." It seemed to me that it would have been very hard for these members to sit in the congregation and hear this, unless they were still proud of their past. One can only assume that he had permission of the former sinners to do this story about them. Anyway, I quit confiding anything to Pastor Larsen after that. The church built a large retirement center on its own property. As I remember, Uncle Carl's family was very active in developing and financing that project. This is where Uncle Carl happily resided in his own retirement until his death.

Schoitz had approximately two hundred beds and was a very nice nonprofit community hospital. It was an easy eight-mile drive from our home in Cedar Falls. It was one of three hospitals in Waterloo and has since merged with St. Francis Hospital, which was about a mile away. The hospital contracted with Midwest Emergency Associates to staff the ER with doctors, and the hospital supplied the other ER personnel. The ER was very nice and well run. There was a full-time nurse manager of the ER, and staffing was adequate. Dr. Singer was my immediate boss, as director of the ER for Midwest Emergency Associates. He worked his share of shifts, something which many in his directorship position did not do. We had a very good relationship, and I kept in touch with Dr. Singer and his family for years.

We worked either twelve- or twenty-four-hour shifts at Schoitz, and I generally enjoyed the work. We had some fun, too. We thought we were busy, but our patient load was nothing like what we'd have in later years. At that time, we were at least able to get some rest on the night shift.

A man in his late twenties came into the ER one evening shortly after I arrived. I believe he had a back complaint. He found out that I had come from the air force, and he indicated that he was an F-15 pilot. We had a nice long conversation about the F-15, and I was so excited to meet someone who could talk with me on my own level about flying. I've forgotten how his case ended, but I'm sure that fellow got whatever he came for. I had not had the experience at that time to be able to recognize a fraud and a manipulator. Only upon looking back years later did I realize that I had been taken. That boy had probably never been near a fighter plane. He must have had a good laugh that night.

We generally saw good salt-of-the-earth-type people in Iowa who actually worked, paid their bills, raised good families, and deserved good care. This was in contrast to the general population seen in Kansas City during my residency and was more what I thought emergency medicine should be like.

Mrs. Moser, from Hudson, was one of my favorite nurses. She and I had one good day in which we felt that we had actually saved two very viable lives. On that day, two men in their fifties came in, only several hours apart, and collapsed in ventricular fibrillation right in front of us. We shocked them both out of their fibrillation and back to normal rhythm and they awakened in the ER. They were admitted, and I believe both were eventually dismissed to go home. This day was special because so many of our "saves" with the defibrillator occur on people so ill or old that it may have been better if they had not been saved.

Another memorable day at Schoitz was when a man about my age (early forties) was brought in unconscious with what turned out to be a large subarachnoid hemorrhage—a stroke or bleed inside the head. I did the initial life-preserving procedures and looked at the chart and name only later when there was time. I was shocked to realize that the patient was someone with whom I'd grown up. Because I knew the family, I did contact them to see if any of the family wanted to do CT studies to see that none of them had the same defect. They did not want any studies and that is okay. Not everyone wants to know. Some don't want the DNA tests either—for this reason or others. The studies may reveal too much to people they don't want to know the findings.

I enjoyed kidding with two young, beautiful, competent night nurses, Pam and Mrs. Larabee. I once made off with another hospital employee who they would not know and had him recline in a room with a sheet over him. I had him play like he was a violent patient. We applied the gag safety-pin-through-the-nose and called the nurses to the room to help me with this "uncooperative" patient. They made considerable effort to calm this poor unfortunate man before realizing that the whole thing was a joke. We could still get away with that kind of nonsense at that time. Later, it would be too risky legally, and besides, there wouldn't be time.

On another occasion, these same two nurses helped embarrass Lyle Sunderman. Lyle and Ardith visited and were taken to see the ER at night when Pam and Mrs. Larabee would be on duty. I arranged for both of these girls to welcome Lyle effusively, as if he were a long-lost and much-missed date. Ardith did not know what to think for a few moments, but it soon became apparent that the welcome was too friendly to be true. This effort did not prove to be as funny as I thought it would. It was just too complicated.

A young man came in one night with a penile abscess. I asked Pam and Mrs. Larabee to assist me, as we needed to incise and take cultures. The man was reclining on the cart, and I realized only later that I did not need to lean over to work on the end of the penis, which is where the abscess was, because the penis was so long. I was so engrossed in my work that I had not noticed this unusual organ length. While discussing the case later with the girls, I was surprised at how I had not even noticed what seemed so rare and unusual to them. I just told them that I thought all were about that length.

Our habit was to put lab samples on the counter to be picked up by the lab. One day at shift change, when the most workers would be there, I poured some Cepacol (which is yellow and looks like urine) into a sterile urine collection bottle and placed it on that counter with the rest of the lab samples. I kept my eye on that bottle very closely, and at the most opportune time, I started acting strangely, drawing as much attention as possible. I grabbed that bottle and drank it. Most, at that moment, were sure I had lost my mind—and it took some explaining to reverse that opinion.

One day, I took the fake disappearing ink to work and had fun spraying folks (fellow workers, not patients) with it. Most of them thought it was totally out of character for me to do something so destructive of personal property, and they would be much relieved when the stains disappeared from their clothing within two minutes. I had learned that with a joke like this, it was better to use it initially among a small group so they could then be involved in playing the joke on others as new suckers either arrived or were selected. I would then enjoy watching others spread the joke. This one backfired big time, though, as some of our ER staff went next door and sprayed the OR crew with the disappearing ink. The OR crew henceforth picked up their ketchup-and-mustard-type bottles of mercurochrome and iodine and sprayed back with huge volumes of liquids, and those did *not* disappear from our ER uniforms.

A big new story while at Cedar Falls was that an ER doctor who worked at another hospital killed his entire family, four children and his wife, in his basement. I passed that house every day on the way to work, and I could not help but think of that each time I drove by. Our ER nurse director later bought and lived in that house. Another news story told of two farmers who died from gasses produced by silage while working down in their silo.

After being in Iowa for several years, we grew restless to move on. Our original plan when leaving general practice was to move every few years so the family could experience various parts of the country and different lifestyles. We planned to do that until they started high school, when it would be better for them to stay put. Doing ER medicine and working for others allowed that plan to work. It was also probably the reason my mother-in-law thought I could not hold a job. The moving was a good thing, and there was an unbelievable pay increase with each move, although some of the older generation in small towns think that anyone who leaves that small town must be defective in some way.

We had decided to get in one more move before settling down and thought it would be fun to live in Hawaii for a year or two. Since I would need to again travel to the location to get the job and then find a place to live, I spent much time in 1979 at the Cedar Falls Library learning about the fiftieth state. I would look at hospitals on Oahu and Maui, so I found some bargain places to stay and marked off ten days of vacation for the trip.

My father, Orval Otte, became more ill shortly before I was to leave, so I cancelled and spent the time with my dad. Having this time off allowed me to be with my dad for his last ten days. He was at University of Nebraska Hospital and diagnosed with primary liver cancer. The doctors had elected not to treat aggressively, as it was too far advanced. Dad said he'd had no alcohol for two years, but I believe the doctors thought that his hepatic symptoms were from resuming alcohol. I truly believe Dad was "dry," but the doctors' assumptions were reasonable, given the usual pattern of alcoholics. I stayed in the visitor's quarters at the hospital and was able to be with him most of the time during the days. He was worse, so I stayed, and on the last day, he died about one o'clock a.m. on March 8, 1979. I remember that sometime during his stay he had wanted me to tell his roommate the story of the burglar who got caught in the chimney in Kansas City. Dad was bedfast due to weakness, and I remember being able to be there to turn him frequently. I also used a hair dryer to dry his skin—all to avoid decubitus ulcers, which he did not get. The care by the hospital staff was outstanding, and we wrote a commendation letter to Dad's hospital floor after the funeral.

Sometime later, on a rainy day in the spring of 1979, we held a sale of the folks' belongings. I remember a Victrola-like machine that played tubular recordings and brought about four hundred dollars. And I wish we would have kept a set of thin red books that Kim expressed an interest in. As I remember, all of the household and farm items brought about twelve thousand dollars.

My trip to Hawaii still took place, but not until later in 1979. The purpose of the trip was to find an ER job so we could experience the islands for several years. I remember going through Frommers and other travel publications to plan the trip and find the best lodging deals. I was so proud when I found a ridiculously low-priced motel in Oahu, which was to be my home base. The flight from LA was my first time to fly over water, and the five hours seemed long. For some reason I was upgraded to first class, which helped. Upon landing, we received the usual lei greeting and I shared a cab with another lady who lived near downtown Honolulu. The cab driver asked my destination. When I told him my motel name, both he and the other passenger doubled over in laughter, but they wouldn't tell me why. It was a little late at night, and I thought it strange that the motel clerk was in a room behind bars. I stayed that one night but heard that they were fumigating the place the next day, so I packed up early and hit the street, on foot, with my suitcases. That first motel apparently was one the locals called a "cat house," so I assume that is the reason for the funny responses in the cab. I found a nice, fairly reasonable hotel within walking distance that morning and was able to start my interviews.

I rented a car on each island and it was pretty inexpensive, since one could not drive far. The islands were beautiful and not so crowded then, but it rained some each day. My best interview on Oahu was at Queen's Hospital, which was the trauma center for all of the islands. I socialized and went to a meeting with the group at Queens. The rest of the group was either Asian or local, and their main concern was whether I would be able to communicate with the locals. I actually received a good job offer from them and did not decline it until I finished the trip and talked it over with Twyla back home.

The doctor on Maui said that I was about the hundredth to apply for the job there and the tenth to visit. I also visited one hospital on the island of Hawaii. Each of the islands had only one or two hospitals at that time. Medicine seemed about ten years behind the rest of the country then, and it seemed the same about five or ten years later when Twyla and I revisited. By the time I visited the last two islands, I realized the pay would be about a third less and expenses about a third more. Our four girls would have had to attend private schools because the locals don't like white kids and do violence to them when they can. I'd heard that they have a "kill a howie day" at school. Private tuition would have cost about ten thousand dollars per child per year. Twyla doesn't really like water, and we weren't sure she would tolerate being so surrounded by it. I was told that some people get "island fever" and are not happy. I also heard that the state requires job applicants to prove that they have the money to get back to the mainland before they are hired. I looked at some of the local residential areas and decided that the islands were well geared to tourists but might not be such a pleasant place to live for the two years that we thought we would stay. Twyla and I reconfirmed that feeling when we visited about five years later. Therefore, we are glad we decided to make the move to Phoenix in 1980.

While in Cedar Falls/Waterloo, I had a job offer from St. Luke's in Phoenix for a slight raise in pay, but I actually received about a thirty percent raise in pay by the time I started work there. We seemed to be stuck on the name "Luke." There was the air base, the dog, and now the hospital, all named Luke. I must read the epistle of Luke sometime.

My contract in Iowa was over in June, so we planned to move to Phoenix and start work there in July. We sold the Lawn Boy lawnmower and Herbie the car to someone from work. The rest of the stuff we didn't want to move was sold at an auction, run by a school principal we knew. My school microscope sold for about twice what we paid for it in 1958. I believe the huge entertainment system we had since La Salle days was disposed of at this time, as we didn't move it to Phoenix. We made flyers and sold the house ourselves. Several estimates were done, and we priced it above those. We had so much activity on the house that we took it off the market and priced it higher and then sold it to a very nice couple whose lawyer drew up the sale documents.

We loved our red and black Dodge van and decided to keep it to use in Phoenix, even though the color on the upper part of the van was black and would not be ideal in the heat and sun of Arizona. We also had lots of winter clothing that we would not use again. Luke (our black poodle) would travel with us in the van to our new home. We all had good friends in Iowa to bid good-bye, and we promised to keep in touch. Uncle Carl and Aunt Ada "sold" us some furniture out of their house for a very low price. The movers therefore, made a stop at their home and loaded a harvest table, a couch, and a hutch. These were quality items and have served our family well. Some will be handed down to our children.

Chapter Ten

Phoenix

1980-1996

We liked a lot of things about Cedar Falls/Waterloo and had many good friends there, but we really did want better weather. Kim, our oldest, would start high school in the fall of 1980, and we wanted to be settled in one place for all four to finish their high school years without moves. I had some great contacts in Phoenix that enabled me to get a good job. Our friend, Dr. Fisher, had worked at St. Luke's Hospital for a year and liked it there. We'd also met Drs. Bursey, Kunkel, Vance, and Ryan at emergency medicine meetings we'd attended while in the air force during the years of 1975–1977.

The Cedar Falls house was sold, the moving van came, and we loaded into the 1979 red and black Dodge van for the move to Phoenix.

I'm sure we went through Clarinda for some last good-byes and then took I-80 west through Greeley, Albuquerque, and Payson on the way to our new home. We stopped in Payson for a meal before the final eighty-mile assault on Phoenix. We left our dog Luke in the car with the windows rolled down a little. Since Luke would bite even friends, we couldn't imagine what he would do to an intruder. Our entire family was having a peaceful meal in an alpine-like restaurant when a frantic lady came in screaming about a dog left in a car out front. She demanded to know to whom the dog belonged and proceeded to lecture us on why one can't leave a dog in the car in Arizona heat. As we know now, she was right, but it was not a very good introduction to the state. She had all the passion of a TV evangelist or a PETA demonstrator.

The kids were excited to see their new home. Twyla and I had been to Phoenix several months before to search out schools and buy a house. We selected the schools first and then found a home in that area. The house was about a year old and was built by a Dial executive who had been relocated. A single ranch-style, four bedroom, three-bath home, it had 2,850 square feet on about one acre. We had paid $180,000 for it with $150,000 borrowed at 11 percent. The front was finished with a few palm trees and about 8,000 square feet of hybrid Bermuda grass. The back was unfinished and was all desert dirt.

Our first several nights were spent on sleeping bags in the new house, as the furniture had not yet arrived from Iowa. The house had been lived in for a year but had been empty for about a month before we arrived. We found several scorpions on the floor at bedtime, and Twyla says that she killed them with a shoe while I cowered somewhere. I don't remember that story as well as Twyla does.

We lived only a few miles from the north edge of town, as it was then. The twenty-four acres just northeast of the Fifty-Fourth and Cholla intersection and our home was raw desert. The usual desert plants and wildlife lived there, including coyotes and jackrabbits. There were plans a few years later for that area to become a Christian high school. The neighborhood rose up to prevent this, and I must say that I was considerably embarrassed at how mean-spirited some of the neighbors were about this. I realize now that they were right to resist that school in the middle of our residential area.

The Palo Verde insect is a black beetle-like bug that can be two- to four inches long. We all stood on the driveway on the north side of our house one night and heard something walking out of the desert from the east. We realized that it was a Palo Verde bug only when we saw it crawl down the curb on the east side of the street and continue toward our garage. I found out later that these bugs defend themselves vigorously when one unwittingly finds one in a gunny sack with one's fingers.

The house at 5349 East Cholla Street (the northeast corner of Fifty-Fourth Street and Cholla) was in Phoenix, but fortunately, it had a Scottsdale mailing address. I understand that if it had been several miles south in Paradise Valley, the value of the house would have been at least fifty thousand more. In 1980, Paradise Valley Mall was just being developed and was about a mile to the northwest of our home. Orange Tree Golf Course was two blocks east of our home. A very nice tennis club would later be built a half mile south at Fifty-Fourth and Shea. The homes already in the area were mostly similar to ours in style and age, with about half to be built after ours, which was built in 1979. The home directly across the street east of ours was built after we arrived. The owner was himself a builder, and he spent the entire four months personally observing all aspects of the build. The home had eight thousand square feet under one roof, some of that being patio. The home had some innovations, one of which was the simple large fans embedded in the ceiling which took the warmer upper air out into the attic. The owner said that his cooling bill for that house was about a hundred dollars per month when ours was about three hundred dollars.

The house described above was occupied by several nice families while we lived there. The last family to live in the house included a man in the high-end food business and catering.

Their boys, of high school and college age, were nice. The father always went to work in a black tuxedo and was picked up by a limousine. When the family moved out, the home was for sale and empty for about a month. One Friday during that time, a young man in his late teens or twenties came to our door. His movements were a little jerky, and he appeared nervous, with poor eye contact. He wanted us to know that his family had purchased the house and that they would hold a party there that night. He wanted us to know so the activity would not bother us so much. At about dusk, cars started arriving and they parked everywhere, including the lanes and both sides of the street for at least a block in each direction from the corner. The crowd, mostly high-school age, was extremely loud and unruly. They congregated all over the street and around the house, easily numbering five hundred or more. I called the previous owner, who said that there was no sale and he knew nothing of the party. He said his son would be over and that I should call the police. When the son arrived, he was confronted by some chain-swinging young men who appeared to be guarding the party. When the police arrived, everyone left quickly. The police said this was a common occurrence and that the group was probably already at another empty house. The party organizers, most likely drug dealers, would identify empty houses for their parties and would get the word out very efficiently, and this was before cell phones. The police said it was fortunate they had not yet gained entrance into the house. When that happened, the partygoers would knock out all the inside walls to have one large room for their activities.

The house directly across from us on the north was occupied initially by a family, also with four boys, of elementary school age. They were a great help to Twyla on the day our house was burglarized. The father was an optometrist, but not practicing in that field. He was into sales of solar hot water and pool units, electric cars, and oil well investments. Being a doctor, he had an "in," so he sold many of his products to physicians. He was not pushy, but he did encourage us to invest five thousand dollars in a new oil well field near Milliken, Colorado. This was of special interest to us since the field was near Greeley, where we lived for the first ten years. We didn't have extra money at that time, but we did go to his office downtown to learn more about the investment. I remember the office being extravagant, housed in one of the high-rise business offices on Central. The name of the investment company, which is long since gone, projected from the wall behind the receptionist in raised gold letters about one foot high and three inches thick. Our neighbor promised that if the oil investment failed, he would give us five thousand dollars' worth of solar hot water product. We still didn't make the investment. That expensive sign, the office, and his two very expensive personal cars bothered us. He never caused us to feel bad about not investing with him. One day, the house was suddenly empty and they were gone, with no goodbyes or forwarding information. The word was that they had taken bankruptcy. I did receive a call from one ophthalmologist who had invested a large sum and really wanted to find our neighbor. One of our girls visited them in Washington State several years later and they were living quite high. He had his expensive sports cars back and they lived in a house with its own elevator. I suspect he was back in the same business. The wife also was very nice. I just hope she doesn't mind moving every three-to-five years.

The above house was then sold to a nice couple who would become our good friends. We were discussing our water bills one night and they noted that theirs was about a tenth of ours. He notified the water company about the discrepancy. They investigated and found that someone had hooked all of the outdoor and pool water plumbing *ahead* of the meter. This was corrected and then their water bills were similar to ours.

These same neighbors had an aunt in a nursing home who was extremely obese and got around in a wheelchair. They were nice enough to bring her to their home for visits and meals occasionally. On one of these weekends, she slipped out of her wheelchair or the car and onto the driveway. Several of our daughters and sons-in-law were home that weekend and were summoned across the street to help get her into some kind of upright position. It must have been quite an experience. When they lifted in one place, the fat would simply roll or slinky somewhere else and she would stay on the ground. They finally accomplished the task, and I suspect their success was due to one of Phil's lifting innovations.

The neighborhood was great for our walking and running. Twyla enjoyed the streets and alleys north of our home and north of Cactus. I would go with her in that area some of the time, but I had several running routes south of the home and through the Orange Tree area. We enjoyed the area so much that even ten years after living there, we'd park the car and cover those routes. After walking one morning, Twyla came back home saying that a lady was in a deep hole in her small red sports car several blocks from our place. Twyla called the report in and I ran up to look. Sure enough, the city had excavated a large hole about twenty feet deep in the middle of Fifty-Second Street, just north of Cholla. An expensive-looking sports car containing an equally expensive-looking Scottsdale lady sat wheels-down in the bottom center of that hole. She didn't appear hurt but was just sitting there in the driver's seat trying to look cool—as if she had intended to do that. She saw me but didn't wave. It had rained some, and maybe she didn't see the barricades around the hole at the speed she was going. Thank goodness it didn't rain a lot or that hole would have rapidly filled with water. Fifty-Second Street drained from a long way north down to Shea. I must have needed to go to work that morning, as I can't believe I didn't get my ladder and try to rescue her—or at least stay around to watch the rescue. That must have been quite a shock to be driving along and suddenly find oneself and one's car in a "grave" big enough to bury a house.

The neighborhood was quite upscale, and I suspect that our net worth would have been about the lowest of any near there in 1980. Larry Sunderman said during one of their visits that he knew he was in a good area when he saw one Rolls Royce pass another Rolls Royce. The area was not immune to crime, however. We kept a three-by-five-foot US flag displayed on the front of our house inside the low fence that was part of the house. That flag was stolen three times. After the second time, we hung the flag with bolts through the grommets, but it was still ripped off, leaving part of the flag still hanging. I could not imagine that anyone who would steal a flag would be worth saving. Thus, there were some elaborate plans in my mind to mechanically capture—and punish—the individual. None of these came anywhere close to passing Twyla's review, so we just let them keep stealing our flag. On another occasion near the end of our stay there we had a drive-by shooting attempt. I was in the garage ready to enter the house when a car went by and fired a shotgun. Four pellets lodged in the doorjamb in front and in the wall behind me. I didn't realize at first what it was and went on into the house where I then thought about the sound from the street and of the pellets hitting nearby. We went back out to look and found the holes and pellets. I believe it was random, as we had no neighborhood enemies. Disgruntled patients from work would be another story, though. We were always proud of being listed in the phone book, but maybe that was not so smart for an ER physician. Twyla, who puts the best construction on everything, never did believe my story and chalked it up to the genetic Otte exaggeration and histrionics.

The garage of our home was a standard two-car size. That meant that one had to squirm sideways to get out of the cars, and with a full-sized van it is even worse. We talked much of building an adequate garage on the west side of the house and converting the current one into a game room. We also dreamed of a covered circle drive. There was a small storage room off to the left as one entered the current garage. It held the water softener, tools, and yard and house chemicals. Our water had a chemical taste, and Kim soon figured out that it was from storing chemicals in the same room as the softener. The water softener had a charcoal feature in it to take taste out of the water. Being in that small room, the charcoal probably absorbed those smells and put them back into the water. When we removed the chemicals from the storage room, the taste went away. I have noted a similar taste in water in some homes, and I wonder how many people don't know to keep the two separated.

The electric water heater was also in that same small room. I drilled holes in the south wall to hang shelving and drilled through a water pipe, requiring a plumber visit. Guess I should be happy that we didn't need an electrician.

We had been hearing good things about solar hot water heaters, and we'd noticed some in the area had the units on their roofs. The units cost about thirty-five hundred dollars, but the federal and state tax rebates paid for all but about three hundred of it, which made it cost about the same as another electric unit to replace our current heater, which had just quit. Being a sucker for gimmicks, I had it installed. The unit consisted of two solar collector panels, about three-by-six foot, and an eighty-gallon insulated storage tank. The water would circulate through the black collectors and be heated by the sun, and the hot water would be stored in the tank. There was a 4,500-watt heater in the tank for the times when there would not be enough sun. The unit seemed to work well, and we had plenty of hot water and lower electric bills. The downside was the appearance of the panels on the roof as well as some yearly maintenance, which I couldn't do. There was a sacrificial rod which needed to be replaced about every three-to-five years. All went well for several years until one Christmas when all twenty-three of the Otte clan visited and stayed with us. We were taking family pictures outdoors when water started to run off the roof. It had been a cold night and the water in the collectors froze and broke the pipes. There were some cold Otte showers that trip. Fortunately, it didn't happen until near the end of their stays.

Either the government or the company paid for most of the replacement cost of the unit with a passive system. In this system, antifreeze circulated through the collectors, and the heat was exchanged to water in the tank, so there was nothing to freeze. The installer had two kinds of collectors—standard and chrome. The chrome cost a hundred dollars more, which we would have to pay. He didn't want to sell them to me, as he said they were too powerful for Phoenix. He was talking to someone who used only the high setting on everything, so you might guess I had to have those. Knowingly, he left a fitted tarp cover for one of the two units. It turned out I had to cover one collector every summer, and even then, boiling water came out the overflow most of the time, so the chrome *was* too strong for Phoenix. The solar hot water heater otherwise worked well during our entire time in that home, and I'm sure it paid for itself many times over.

Twyla's slow and careful driving was legend during those school years. I worried that someone would get upset sometime following her. Combine that with the fact that the girls thought it was funny to extend the fourth (ring) finger with the least provocation.

The girls all had work assignments around home on weekends. Pat and Pam were helping me wash the van one Saturday. They were at the back of the van when they both broke out into uncontrolled laughter. They had found feathers and "bird grease" all over, so mother had obviously had a bird strike *on the back window*. We knew that would be hard to get unless the bird was flying faster than she was going.

My original 1980 Honda eventually got so that it wouldn't climb the hills to Payson where I did some work at that time. When I got my new 1987 blue Honda Accord, I was very proud of and happy with it. One Saturday, Twyla and I had gone somewhere in the old red-and-black Dodge van. The girls knew how important a clean car was to me, so they scrubbed down my new car with steel wool soap pads. It really didn't do any damage, but you can imagine how unappreciative I was of their work. It turned out all right, but the girls still remember the event.

I got caught once by two motorcycle cops, a half block south of our garage, doing forty-five in a thirty-five-mile-per-hour zone. That was when I was going to work in the old 1980 Honda. I guess it didn't do any good that I told them that car couldn't *do* forty-five in a half block. I didn't challenge it any further, and reluctantly attended a good driving school for eight hours. My birthday was soon after that, and Twyla and the girls made a birthday cake showing me behind bars on top of the cake.

Another 1980 Honda episode was when the car floated through a flood. I was on the way to work at St. Luke's in heavy rain. An underpass on Squaw Peak Parkway looked flooded, so I stopped a little way back to see if cars were making it through and whether traffic was backing up behind me. It appeared that traffic was moving, so I got back on the road and then was committed, with traffic coming behind me. It was evident upon getting closer that no one was going out the other side of the water and were, in fact, all sinking to the roadway in my way. I floated backward past a pickup, with the lanes ahead blocked by sunken cars. The only way past was around the other side of that pickup on the inside lane, which was still open. I knew that the Honda was floating because when I looked out the window I was looking down into the bed of that pickup. I pushed some on the gas, and much to my surprise, that stopped the backward drift and gave enough control to go back behind that pickup and then forward into that inside lane. I was able to maneuver among the sunken cars and out the distal side of that water and I kept going on to work. The water had been three or four feet deep, but no one was in imminent danger, as it was accumulated water, not rushing water. A small amount of water had come into the passenger compartment, so once I got to work, I parked on the steepest hill I could find so the water could drain out. We had to replace a water pump some time later, probably because of the moisture, but otherwise the Honda continued to do well.

There was a sign on Shea Boulevard that said, "Horse for Sale," and we just got used to it. Larry noted one time that that horse had been for sale for fourteen years, and he wondered what shape it was in.

Our house had a predominantly flat tar roof which began leaking at about three years. We applied a white foam material that appeared to have good insulating qualities and did not leak. Some low areas held water, as the roofers said that they could not get the slope such that all the water would drain. I always thought they should have been able to fix that.

We found a gooey substance on the north wall of the dining room one day. Further examination outdoors showed a hole at about ceiling level with lots of bee activity. We had them exterminated and the hole in the outer wall sealed. We've talked to others who had the same problem. Many of them had to tear into the walls to remove the honey from inside. Fortunately, we didn't need to do that, so we think the hive hadn't been there long. Later, one other swarm attached itself to a corner of the patio roof and had to be removed. This was all before the time of the killer bees.

Twyla was walking on the tile floor in the kitchen one Sunday morning when she noted that the tile was warm. This led us to discover a hot water leak under the cement slab under the family room. If it had been cold water, I don't know how long it would have taken to discover. Repair of this required taking up the carpet in the family room, breaking through the cement slab, and finding the crimped copper pipe. We had a good plumber who was able to find and break through the cement right over the leak. That pipe must have sustained a ninety-degree bend sometime during installation. We disclosed the event before the sale of the house, and I understand that the new owners had another leak sometime later, also under that family room.

We'd had a tremendous amount of water under the house with the above event, so much that the insurance company did some examination under the support walls and found they were okay. We had no more hot tile, but six weeks later we did have termites. Because termites need a dependable source of water, those trails they build are so that they can get outdoors to that water source. Twyla saw little "trails" hanging from the ceiling in the entryway, and we had the full termite treatment for a thousand dollars. I have been very compulsive since then about keeping water away from the house foundation.

The house had four bedrooms. Kim, probably because she was the shortest, got the smaller middle bedroom halfway down the hall, known as the rainbow room. Valerie got the waterbed room, leaving the larger room off the kitchen that had the blue carpet for Pat and Pam.

The kitchen was small for the size of the house, but Twyla prepared many successful meals there. The garbage disposal in the sink was super strong and would grind up a horse, and it did grind many citrus rinds. The mixer built into the countertop was powerful and made many margaritas.

The family room was used for a lot of parties and post-event gatherings while the girls were in high school and college. It had custom-made oak shelving and cabinets, some of which held the 32-inch TV and the sound system. It eventually held laser vision and surround-sound systems of which I was proud and which everyone else tolerated. It was state-of-the-art for that time. The small wet bar at the back of the room was not used much.

We thought the sunken living room was not too useful, and that it would have been nice if it had been combined with the family room. The people who bought the house in 1977 did attempt to combine the two rooms by using a large beam to replace the weight-bearing wall between them.

My three sisters, Irma, Vera, and Ruth surprised me on my fiftieth birthday in 1986. I had just finished a twenty-four-hour shift on the morning of their arrival. Twyla put me to bed after feeding me well, I'm sure, and telling me she was going out to get groceries. Instead, she went to the airport to pick up the sisters. She brought them home where they went to the "blue room" in the other end of the house and changed into black dresses complete with veils and gloves. They then went out to the front door and rang the doorbell. Twyla answered the door, then awakened me and said some religious people were at the door that she couldn't get rid of. I told her to put the chain on our dog Buddy's collar and Buddy and I would go to the door. Twyla had set the video camera on a tripod and had it running from a far corner. Buddy and I opened the door and sure enough, there were three women in black singing a dirge song which I didn't recognize as "happy birthday" until they got to the "happy birthday dear brother" part. I don't believe I've ever been so surprised—except when the twins were born. Ruth and Vera had wanted to dress in Clarinda and come on the plane that way, but Irma would have no part of that. The first thing they did after my surprise was to put me back to bed and then they went *shopping*. Paradise Valley Mall had some special event that day with lots of helium-filled balloons. The girls asked a security guard if they could have some of the balloons to help their brother celebrate his birthday and he said, "Sure, ladies, you can have anything you want." They filled that red-and-black van with those balloons to the point that I'm surprised it stayed on the ground. They then arranged the balloons in a big half circle on the front of the house with a large happy birthday banner across the middle. We have videos of that and of playing with the balloons in the pool the next day. Since Twyla had assisted in the arrangements, the visit came at a time when I was off duty, so we had three or four days of a great time.

Our four girls were in their late grade school and early high school years when we moved to Scottsdale in 1980. It was a time when we expected they'd make use of a nice backyard, so we elected to not wait until we could afford to finish the backyard but to borrow the money and do it early. So within about a year of moving in, we borrowed the extra fifty-five thousand and started the work. We had definite ideas of what we wanted, and Dale, our landscaper, drew up plans. Since the girls had been into swimming in Iowa, we wanted a pool long enough for them to do laps. We had seen sunken tennis courts at the tennis clubs and liked that idea too. We wanted lots of lighting and plants that would bear fruit. Since the lot was a commercial acre, there would be just enough room for all of that.

This next section will be about our experiences in building the backyard. I've often said that I should write a book about that project.

As a reminder, we were from Iowa, where you can trust that people will do what they promise, but here it was not to be so.

First, we contracted for the pool after extensive shopping. It would be forty feet long, a little longer than most, so as to allow lap swimming. There would be a porpoise-like cleaner which would simply run about stirring up the dust so that it could be taken off through the diatomaceous earth filter. We had originally planned to have solar heating for the spa, but we changed that to gas heat, for an extra cost, when we figured out that solar would heat the water only during the daytime and would extend the swimming season by only a few weeks on each end. The gas heater was sized to be able to heat the entire pool at any time, which we did often during the Christmas holidays. There were nice steps in the pool and an area on each side to sit in the water. We chose brown tile to better match the house. The depth was increased by several feet to allow a diving board. But the building of the pool needed to wait until completion of the tennis court.

We contracted for the tennis court with a local company that had done many courts in the area, including those at the nearby tennis club. The company was run by a father and his son Joe, and they indicated they had experience with sunken courts in Michigan where they had come from. A ten-foot fence is standard for a court, and the backyard already had a six-foot fence surrounding the entire yard. By digging down four more feet, we could accomplish the ten-foot fence height. We would then not have to put up a ten-foot fence, which would have certainly bothered the neighbors and would never have been approved. The front-to-back depth of the yard was just enough to allow standard court length. We elected not to light the court, as that would require taller lights which could bother others and would require written permission from neighbors. I had always thought that we might sometime put fluorescents along the top of the fence on the inside, if we found that we used it enough at night. I envisioned steps along about a third of the east side to provide both access to the court and seating. As we would be digging down four feet about a foot inside the yard's wall, we would need to have a fairly strong retaining wall built, which would make up the bottom four feet of our ten-foot tennis court wall. Most of the block to our west drained naturally into our yard, so we needed to make provision for that rainwater to reach Fifty-Fourth Street along the east side of our property. There was a planter about one foot wide, two feet deep, and four feet high between the original yard wall and the new four-foot retaining wall. That water from the rest of the block would come through perforations in the bottom of the yard fence into a cement catchment and be taken by six-inch perforated plastic pipe around the south side of the court, under the soil in the planter. It would then be deposited out into the sump pump collection area, which was a fifty-gallon barrel buried in the southeast corner of the court. As it turned out, there were only a few times any water came into that system, but we still had to provide for it. The plan was for all of the water from the court and whatever came from the rest of the block to be pumped up to a river rock stream which would take the water out to the street. I know this sounds complicated, but it was a sound plan and worked well. Keeping a sump pump working down in that "well" took some effort at times, but it was doable.

The standard tennis court size is 60' x 120', and digging down four feet produces a lot of dirt. The court builders could not keep up with hauling the dirt away, so it accumulated as a huge pile in the rest of the backyard. Some of the neighbors asked us if we were building our own mountain. That "mountain" stayed there for nearly six months. About that time, we began to realize that they would do the next step of the project only when we bugged them. The four-foot wall around the massive hole was built over "L" shaped rebar for strength and stability. The small part of the "L" was at the bottom facing inward, under dirt and the court surface. The surface was to be drained by a one-foot rock-filled moat all around the outer edge, at court level. The builders apparently forgot about that drainage system until after the court surface was poured, but they said they would figure some way to still do that. I came home several days later and found cement cutters with their diamond-tipped circular saws trying to cut out that one-foot section all around the court. They were just starting, but they noted that the rebar under the surface was giving trouble. I stopped them, because those bars were to give stability to the retaining wall of the court. The court was slanted to drain to the sump pump in the southeast corner anyway, so we decided to allow that as the only drainage—and it did work out very well. I found myself getting more involved in the engineering decisions after that. The next problem was that Joe wasn't confident the four-foot retaining wall would stand. We got three written engineering opinions and several unofficial consults. None of them seemed acceptable, so we did what I suggested, which was to pour about three feet of solid cement into the one-foot space between the back side of the retaining wall and the dirt wall under the original fence. The top of that cement stopped about one foot below the top of the retaining wall and was adequate to hold dirt for the planter. The wall has not moved now for twenty-four years and the planter grew some very nice plants.

The six-inch drain tube that was to bring water from the rest of the block to the sump pump ran buried at the bottom of the planter on the south side. It then came around the southeast corner and into the buried fifty-gallon barrel under the court from the east. I came home one night and found a six-inch hole in the east wall above the sump pump area. It looked terrible and ensured we would always have had a dirty path down to the court. I explained the plan to them again. When I came home the next day, I found another hole about two feet lower, but still through the wall. On the third try, they dug it down and brought the tube into the barrel underground without cutting through the wall. They did patch the first two holes in the wall.

We had both a water line and a telephone line that ran down to the slab on the east side of the court. This was long before cordless or cell phones. A basketball hoop was incorporated into the court on the north end. The tennis net was held up by metal and plastic posts that could be extended to hold a volleyball net at its proper height. We probably used the volleyball setup more than the tennis.

The west side of the court was right up against Silverstein's fence. Because the dirt was shaved down right up to that fence, with the exposure of even a portion of the footings, some cracking occurred in one section of their side of the fence. The Silverstein's side of the fence was stucco but not painted. I asked our court builders to fix that problem for the Silversteins. Two attempts were made to have the area re-stuccoed, and it did not match. Apparently, there was some confrontation, as Dr. Silverstein called me, somewhat upset, and asked that Joe and his dad not ever talk to them again. I then took over that part of the project myself. The stucco jobs done on the Silverstein's fence did not match and looked like a cheap patch job. I asked a third group to try to stucco that area and again it failed to match their original stucco. Stucco must be like cement in that each batch looks different. The technique of application is also different for each person.

I then got the Silverstein's permission and hired a good painter to paint the entire inside of their fence to match their house. This solved the problem, as the patches were not visible through paint. I am glad we managed a good resolution, as the Silversteins have turned out to be some of our dearest friends. They are the only neighbors from the Cholla house with whom we have kept in contact, including attending each other's family celebrations. Our four girls are now invited to many of their events also. Our girls babysat for them often, and Valerie had a standing job on Saturday nights with them for some time.

The east side of the court had no wall except for about ten feet of low wall on each end. There was a 8' x 12' cement pad just off the east side of the court in its middle with steps about four feet wide coming off that up to pool level. The soil on either side of the steps sloped gradually to the east up to yard level, providing surface for some nice ground cover.

Anchor Pool Company got to work next and, because of the delays with the court, we started the pool about six months later than planned. The pool was placed about ten feet from the back patio and cool deck filled in all the way around the pool, connecting the pool to the house. The installation went well, and the quality seemed good. I'm glad, because the company was out of business a year later.

Dale and his landscape crew finally got their turn. They installed several more patches of grass and some palms around the pool. Then they planted almost a dozen citrus trees and ran watering to all the areas where I thought I might want more, as well as all the way around the court inside that planter. Dale encased about a 12' x 20' area for a garden along the back wall of the yard. A functioning potential stream with river rock was placed running from the southeast corner of the court out to the street. The "headwaters" of this stream accepted the flow that was brought up from the court by the sump pump.

I initially planted some Iowa-like types of fruit, but they didn't do nearly as well as citrus. We eventually had about twenty citrus trees of the various types I wanted. We saw that two types of citrus in Japan seemed to do well, and we tried these, very successfully. One was an Algerian tangerine that had a "slip peel" and made good eating. Another was a novelty tree (Chandler Pumello) with fruit literally the size of volleyballs. These were very edible if one didn't mind doing some peeling. Because of my propensity for wanting the biggest, best, or most successful, we, of course, had a Ponderosa lemon tree which could make two-pound lemons. That tree is so busy making lemons during most of the year that it just doesn't grow very large.

Much to Twyla's distress, I always had a large compost pile in that garden. Most anything will compost in Arizona if you just put it in a pile and give it some water. Household refuse and many citrus rinds were buried, mostly at posthole depth, so as not to cause an odor. That garden area would have had good compost to about a four-foot depth. I planted something most years but eventually decreased my gardening due to time constraints—and the garden area was filled with my compost-making. The house has sold several times since we lived there, and I see that the present owners took out the garden and have covered the area with sand.

We had some kind of citrus from November through June each year. I purposely picked varieties that would mature at different times, so as to have a long season. Citrus trees produce fruit for a longer time, unlike most of the Midwestern fruits that have short bearing times. It was fun to have company and be able to have them pick as much as they wanted to take back home. One year we picked the excess and took the fruit to a Lutheran nunnery off Fortieth and Shea. One day a man stopped while I was working on the trees and asked if I minded if he picked some fruit for his family to eat. He seemed sincere and nice enough, so I said it was all right. Later that day I looked out and saw people all over, stripping the trees of fruit. He had gone home and brought back two carloads of family or friends. They were picking very fast and I had to ask him to stop. If we had not been home or had not seen them, they would have done some real damage to that year's crop. I'm sure they did this same show repeatedly for a living, with no overhead.

A small seedling palm tree, about six inches tall, sat just outside the entrance to the backyard off Fifty-Fourth Street which was being run over by equipment on the first day of the backyard work. We moved it to the corner of the fence near the garage. It grew to be a full twenty-foot tree and was costing us twenty-five dollars every six months to have it trimmed in later years.

The watering and lighting systems for fully landscaped one-acre yards are quite extensive, and it makes me sick now to even thing about keeping all of that up. There were fifteen valves in those underground boxes connected to timers on the house which ran the drip system. Each plant had to have its own dripper or drippers, all on timers and volume-controlled by the various emitters. A drip system ran all the way around the court in the planter. That system produced some beautiful bougainvillea, pyracantha, and rosemary. None of these would attach naturally to the wall, so they had to be tied to the wall to keep any semblance of order. I spent days on top of that four-foot inner wall, keeping those plants alive, trimmed, and tied up. We had lighting on each plant, and it was beautiful at night. All those lights required upkeep and timers. This was all before LED bulbs, so the electric bill for lighting that yard had to have been big.

I tried at least six times to hire someone to do the care of the landscaping. The first visit would always be good, and then successive visits went rapidly downhill. They wanted a monthly contract, but after a while one would hardly be able to tell that they had been there. I am continually surprised at how good these employees are at appearing very knowledgeable; being so precise at what should be done that one would think their way was the only reasonable way of doing things. They say what has been done previously is always "bad" and that no one else knows how to do it right. They do the things that will make the most show in the shortest time. Some just trim trees with a hedge trimmer and love to use blowers to clean the ground. They learn from work experience what people want to hear and how to impress them. There's no reason to think that they would have done any study about proper trimming or plant diseases. If they lose a job, they can just go to another. For these reasons, I did most of our own yard upkeep and care. I enjoyed trimming and training the citrus to guide the growth and allow easier access to the fruit. There were about ten palm trees on the property which, initially, I could trim. In later years, the trees needed trimming by palm tree trimming specialists at twenty-five dollars per tree every six months. There are groups separate from the general landscapers who have the equipment—and the nerve—to climb the trees and do the trimming. Scorpions love palm trees. Other than falling, there seems to be at least one death each year from palm fronds breaking loose and smothering the trimmer.

I remember that our family once went to a nursery to shop. While there, we noted a lone Don Juan rose in a small pot. We fell in love with it and took it home, planting it on the fence just east of the gate into the backyard near the garage. It flourished and provided us with many beautiful red roses, both outdoors and inside in vases, for our remaining years there.

Because it was so difficult to keep our four girls in house keys (as well as gas caps), we installed a number punch lock in the front door to replace the key system. It seemed, however, that every kid in the high school eventually knew the combination.

The family room had a slanted roof held up by dark brown rafters. We found out that changing that color to an off white required three coats of paint. It really did lighten the room, though, and we liked the change. Pam and I painted the outside of the house and the entire ten-foot-high fence, much of it requiring paint on both sides, during one of her summers off college. We had a bid of eight hundred dollars for painters to do the house. We did it ourselves and put on a thousand dollars' worth of paint alone—in two coats. The prior color had been quite dark, and I wonder if painters would have done two coats. That amount of paint covered the house *and* fence. We figured that the fence area was as much as two more houses. We bought and operated spray-painting equipment and learned a lot in the process. We went back to get more paint and supplies so many times that the guy in the paint store assumed, incorrectly, that Pam liked him.

There were no windows on the west side of the house, but it was covered by a plant that attached itself firmly to the stucco and provided great sun protection. It grew rapidly and profusely but needed trimming often so as not to look too shabby, and we were thankful it shielded the hot sun from that side.

I figure that we had about eight thousand square feet of hybrid Bermuda grass that needed mowing once or twice a week for eight months of the year. It all had to be watered with in-ground sprinklers on timers, and the grass needed lots of water. The sprinklers required frequent repair, replacement, or adjusting. Bermuda must be cut very short, a half inch to an inch, as opposed to Midwest grasses which are cut about two inches high and which don't survive in Phoenix. The Bermuda goes dormant around October and won't come back until the soil temperature warms to sixty degrees in the spring. We brought our nice new rotary mower from Iowa, and it went about two feet in the Bermuda and quit. We learned that one needs a very powerful and expensive reel mower to cut Bermuda. All that watering created lots of thatch, so verti-cutting was required once per year and it was always a surprise how much material would be raised by that procedure. It is possible to have nice green grass year-round in Phoenix, like the golf courses do, if one sews annual rye seed around October. Rye is more like bluegrass and is beautiful. We tried rye for several years and then decided that four months of brown grass wasn't so bad after all, as we'd have a break from seeding, mowing, and watering.

The job that brought us to Phoenix was at St. Luke's Hospital at Eighteenth Street and Van Buren—just east of downtown. Having this job secured allowed us to borrow the money for the home. St. Luke's was an eight-story-high, two-hundred-bed general hospital without pediatrics or obstetrics and had only a level two trauma designation. It had another two hundred newer beds on the south side designated for detoxification from drugs and alcohol and for psychiatric admissions. Most of the cardiac surgery (e.g. bypasses) in Phoenix were done at St. Luke's in those days. The hospital was also known for its poison control center and had three of the nation's fifty board-certified toxicologists on staff. These three areas provided much of the interesting or entertaining happenings about which I write.

Emergency Medicine was still in its infancy in 1980, and I may well have been the only residency-trained and board-certified ER physician in Phoenix at that time. Except for the Luke AFB hospital, I had worked only at "full service" emergency departments that could handle everything and needed to send very little out to other facilities. It was always difficult for me to accept the fact that we could not do everything at St. Luke's, and that is probably part of the reason I usually had a part time job at other emergency departments. I was also fearful of losing my skills in those uncovered areas, and this was a real threat. I must say that St. Luke's was always very good to keep me on full time, even while I was doing part time work at other ERs or exploring other opportunities. I frequently had a job-and-a-half or even two full-time jobs. With four girls in school, we needed the money.

The arrangement at St. Luke's was that the emergency doctors worked directly for the hospital. Most hospitals contracted with ER physician *groups*, and still do. Our arrangement made us, individually, more directly responsible to the hospital. The hospital paid for a full-time administrator/doctor, so we functioned somewhat as a group anyway. That doctor's full-time job was to interface with the hospital and handle the politics, of which there was much. Two ER physicians were always on duty—one in the ER and the second in-house. The in-house doctor's job was to evaluate sudden changes in a patient's condition and provide care until the attending could be contacted or could take over the event. They would also run in-house "codes" (code blues) when a patient went into cardiac arrest.

We in-house doctors were a great source of stability for the nurses. We even started intravenous lines for them when they couldn't. They liked having a physician available immediately who was accustomed to diagnosis, treatment, and procedures associated with end-of-life events. St. Luke's was doing up to five open-chest surgeries daily in the early eighties, and a certain number of these would have complications requiring immediate care. There could be internal bleeding or cardiac tamponade, a life-threatening event. In cardiac tamponade, blood would accumulate inside the sac around the heart until the heart could suddenly no longer pump. The patient would die within minutes unless the chest was reopened and the blood removed or drained. The sutures, including the wire holding the sternum together, would be cut, and at that point the patient might hopefully awaken. The patient would have been unconscious to that point due to their near-death condition. There would be no time for anesthesia, so we gave loads of morphine intravenously so that the patient could be relatively comfortable until they could be moved to surgery for full anesthesia and repair of the bleed by the surgeon. Most of the surgeons lived at least a half hour away.

A "code blue" meant the patient (or visitor or employee) was trying to die and needed immediate intervention. Once the heart stops beating, there is a window of only about five minutes max to re-establish function without permanent damage or confirmed death. A team of about ten people were responsible for responding to that overhead page. These would be nurses or technicians who could provide expertise of any kind or supplies or meds that might be needed. The in-house doctor was responsible for orchestrating the code. This would frequently involve defibrillation (shocking), intubations, and meds, as needed. The in-house doctor was responsible for giving all the orders and deciding when to terminate efforts if there was no response. This decision would take some rapid assessment of information from those who knew something about the patient.

Usually there was not time to depend upon the chart for decision-making. Attendings would not come into the hospital or attend the code on their patient unless they happened to be in the building. Even if they did appear, they frequently wanted us to continue. I once had five successful codes in one day, which must be a record. Dr. Ryan, our boss, decided to play with my mind a little over this. She had an official-looking certificate of appreciation and a badge made up, indicating that they were from administration. I bought into it, thinking the hospital finally realized the value of our services to them, and I was kind of proud to have had a part in that realization. She had to tell me it was a joke before I embarrassed myself even more. Work load for the in-house doctor was sometimes spotty, which allowed us to help out in the ER where we were usually behind. At other times we would go twelve- to twenty-four hours in-house without stopping and would ourselves be behind. We would then have to triage the calls in our minds so that the most urgent were answered first. We spent a considerable amount of our time in the intensive care unit (ICU).

When the attending requested a direct admission for a patient, we in-house doctors would be asked to evaluate the patient first. We would evaluate their orders and make sure the patients were stable enough to wait to be seen by the doctor on his or her next rounds. St. Luke's did not yet have hospitalists to care for inpatients in place of their office doctors. Thus, we were the only doctor to have placed eyes on those admits, for up to twenty-four hours of time. I always thought this practice was a little dangerous for us as well as the patients, and that we were letting their attendings off a little easy. I guess it was somewhat similar when we saw patients in the ER and wrote holding orders for their doctors until they would be seen the next day. We had actually evaluated those patients and participated in their care, so we knew a little more about them. Most doctors did not come in to see their admitted patients unless we asked, or they needed an emergency procedure specific to their specialty.

One of the reasons I went into emergency medicine initially was to give some relief to doctors in practice. My practice in Greeley was so large and I was so conscientious that we moved as close as possible to Weld County Hospital. I would run over many times some nights to the ER to see my patients, as I did not trust the interns to see them. I reasoned that providing quality care by trained ER specialists instead of interns would be a good thing. It seemed logical that if we needed a specialist anywhere, it should be in the ER, where the correct split-second decision could often be the difference between life and death. It made no sense that the sickest and most injured patients were being cared for by interns, the most inexperienced doctors of all. God help them if one arrived in the ER on July 1 when the new batch of interns was starting. I reasoned that the specialty of emergency medicine was badly needed, both for the patients and their doctors, and that it would relieve the doctors of some of the stress that I had felt in practice in 1973. It seemed that it would be a win–win situation for everyone.

I should have known what would happen with such idealism. Look how welfare and other entitlement programs feed upon themselves. It's the old "give 'em an inch and they'll take a mile" behavior. It rapidly got so that office doctors did not plan to see any of their patients after hours, even if they were sick enough to need admission. The doctors—and often their schedulers—sent any overflow to the ER, not wanting to be at risk of staying past closing time. Most city doctors do no suturing, casting, or anything messy in their offices.

I saw a patient in the ER once who had seen his office doctor that morning. When he asked his doctor what he should do if he got worse, the doctor told him to wait until five o'clock and then go to the ER. Another patient was sent to the ER once for an injection, reporting that the doctor had quit giving shots in his office. In my twenty-eight years in the ER, I had opportunity many times daily to talk with doctors or their office staff. I almost always came away from the call with the feeling that the office was crushed with patients, and I almost felt bad for calling them. My feeling was the exact opposite on the times that I would leave the busy, smelly ER to actually go to an office. The offices mostly smelled good and appeared to be pleasant work environments, with little sense of urgency and very few patients visible. An ENT (ear, nose, and throat) doctor once sent us a nosebleed from his office. If he couldn't get it stopped, how could he expect us to accomplish that? That was his specialty. He could have at least come in with the patient to help us. With the above change in doctor behavior, the increased number of uninsured along with a growing population and more trauma, it is no wonder that we have an ER crisis. We have had one for at least twenty years.

The patients have also contributed to the crisis and frustration of ER workers. The world's most needy people are seen almost exclusively in the ER, because the offices won't put up with them. The uninsured and underinsured get much of their primary care in emergency rooms—again, because offices don't have to see them. Many of these folks lead lives of deceit and manipulation. That's what they have to do to survive. They get very adept at knowing when to come and what to say in order to get the care they want at the time they want. You and I (as patients who might have legitimate emergencies) have to compete with the above behavior to have our needs addressed. The addicts are another class entirely and make up at least ten percent of all ER visits. They are champions at the above disruptive behavior. The ER personnel have to sort through all of this behavior constantly, making life-and-death triage decisions and still trying to be fair and nonjudgmental.

The government contributes to the dysfunction by passing an *unfunded* mandate that all who present to an ER have to be evaluated and not triaged away, no matter how trivial the complaint. This legislation was well-meaning and looks good on paper. The triage decision falls to the doctor, and there are heavy fines—fifty thousand against the doctor and another fifty thousand against the hospital—if someone is unstable or is sent away inappropriately. The ER doctor cannot afford to just eyeball the patients, which is the way the designers of the legislation must have thought things were being done. The doctor has to prove beyond a doubt that the patient is okay to be sent away to go to the next office visit that they can get into. The ER doctor is being asked to practically guarantee that the patient will not die or be damaged by waiting to be seen by an outside doctor. The same legislation addresses transfers of patients to other hospitals— along with the same fines. A transfer is not legal if the current hospital has the ability and resources to care for that patient. Thus, the transfer has to be to a higher level of care and the receiving hospital must agree to accept. As you might expect, there is a volume of paperwork associated with a transfer in order to explain our reasoning and, hopefully, to protect us and the hospital where we are working. We make those decision in the heat of trying to care for multiple patients, many of them seriously ill. It is difficult to take time for the necessary documentation when the ER is so backed up, which is the usual case anymore. We make those decisions quickly while our care is fragmented among all the other cases that we have in progress. The government lawyers can take all the time they want to second-guess our decisions, one at a time. If you have read this paragraph thoughtfully, you must be wondering why anyone would want to expose themselves to all this stress and financial risk. Oh yes, besides, it is illegal for the doctor to carry insurance to protect against these government fines. Malpractice insurance cannot cover it, so any fines and defense expenses come directly out of the doctor's pocket. Office practices are not exposed to any of this and can see or decline to see whomever they want. The ER is the only medical entity that *has* to see all comers. Doctors who are called to the ER to see their patient or who accept unassigned ER patients for care within their specialty are also subject to these government mandates and can be fined. Because of this, emergency departments are having more trouble filling call lists of doctors who are willing to take their turn at ER call for their specialty. For a while, hospitals could make being on ER call a condition of staff membership. With the advent of more—and better— outpatient care facilities, many of the specialists can operate their entire practices in those facilities and don't need to use a hospital. This avoids the distasteful ER call and having to care for that type of patient. They thus avoid the mandate that requires them to see all who come, and they can limit their practices to nice people who pay their bills. I truly don't understand how hospitals can afford to have ERs anymore and, indeed, some have quit.

Lawyers are the third reason for the crisis in the ER. When they take a case, they have all the time they might need (and probably one case at a time) to second-guess the ER caregiver. They can shop until they find a "specialist" who will testify for their side. These out-of-state "specialists" do lots of testifying, such that it has become almost a specialty for them. They are paid very well, and the malpractice attorney also takes a third to a half of any award the patient wins. I understand that the doctor wins 90 percent of cases that go to jury, but many cases are settled before that, for a variety of reasons. For the malpractice attorney, it's "all in a day's work," but for the doctor it is a devastating experience. The doctor has to spend a considerable amount of his time in preparation of his defense and in depositions and testifying. The *only* person in this whole process not being paid for his efforts is the doctor being sued—even if he wins. Any doctor with any kind of conscience will suffer severely at the accusing, degrading nature of the case. The stress is hard on family life and marriage. A malpractice case surely shortens the life of the doctor, and for this reason, I consider that malpractice lawyers are doing a little murder all throughout their careers. Emotional "show-biz" tactics, along with questionable jury selection procedures as well as entrapment tactics against the defendant and his witnesses and magnification of the importance of certain opinions and articles that would support his contentions are all part of his unsavory game. For these reasons I believe that lawyers should be taken entirely out of the malpractice game (and that is the way they look at it—as a game) and be replaced by a commission of professionals who would evaluate the cases quickly, without the theatrics. The patient does need protection from true mistakes and bad doctors, and the commission could be empowered to make judgments and awards. It would not be without some mistakes, but it can't be worse than what we have now. This group or groups would do this job professionally and full time. They are much more likely to see patterns and be better able to weed out or restrict the doctors who practice poor medicine. The court costs and lawyer fees would be eliminated, and awards would be fair, without the threat of the unreasonable windfalls we have now.

Enough of the serious stuff. The reason for writing all of this is to entertain and maybe inform a little. As I started to write, I realized that the rest of life also had some interesting tales, so what was to be an

ER book got expanded. There are so many strange and unusual happenings in the ER that I want to share some before I forget them.

***

I don't remember my first day at St. Luke's, but I do know that they provided a week of double coverage so a new person could become accustomed to the routine before they would be on their own. No other hospital had done that. St. Luke's ER had six rooms and eight or nine beds during most of my time there. Initially that was adequate, but as business in all ERs picked up—for the reasons spoken of above—more beds were required. My only goal was to be the best emergency physician that I could be, and I was not interested in the financial or administrative positions. That doesn't mean I did not have definite ideas about how an ER should function. Poor Dr. Bursey (our administrative doctor) would receive two or three pages of suggestions from me. He would initiate a few of the suggestions, but usually nothing that would cost very much. The ER had full-time doctors for at least five years before I arrived. Most of these doctors had quit their local practices to do only ER work at St. Luke's. I finally learned over the years that administrators do not really appreciate suggestions and want to keep things status quo.

We usually had one or two nurses and sometimes one tech on at a time, and I thought that was inadequate much of the time. They were often busy checking patients in or out and could not be available to the doctor to assist them in a timely manner.

St. Luke's was into being a base station for fire department paramedics. Some of them were trained at St. Luke's with their six-month courses. The paramedics were very well trained, but still had to call the St. Luke's ER doctor if they were going to give any treatment on the street. These calls were frequent and would disrupt what we were doing. If we were gloved for a procedure, we would have to take the call and re-glove. The paramedics knew their business, and I seldom felt I had added anything to their care.

I will quit complaining now. These were some of the frustrations with emergency medicine in general and with the work conditions. Each ER had various quirks which I thought could be improved upon, but I was not the administrator. It was difficult for someone as compulsive as I am to work within systems that I thought could be more efficient.

Louise had been the night nurse at St. Luke's ER since long before I arrived on the scene. She was a very good nurse and had saved my butt many times. I have always said that I needed to be good to Louise because if she talked, I would be ruined. We had a considerable bit of fun at work in the early years, but in later years that would have been too risky. Maybe it was because I was getting older and we were busier. Louise was of adequate size and had a no-nonsense face. She was the only nurse during the 11:00 p.m. to 7:00 a.m. shift, and she hated having drunks occupy her beds through the night. Soon after coming on for her night shift, Louise would make her rounds. She would identify the drunks, throw their covers off, and put her face right over them, announcing "Time to go home." These folks may not have had a home, but they knew that they wouldn't be spending the night in Louise's ER bed. She was very accurate in her evaluations, and we never got in any trouble over it. St. Luke's ER was downtown in a bad area, so it was always nice to have a few beds empty for nighttime emergencies. We were not supposed to get the severe traumas, but sometimes they would come anyway because of our location.

A clerk always stood near the swinging doors of the entrance to check patients in. She would have the patients sit while asking the required information. This took a while, and over the years this duty grew in volume, as did all other documentation. One night a man in his thirties was being checked in and I noted him sitting on only one hip. He was sitting that way because he had fallen in the shower and "wouldn't you know it" a shampoo bottle that was sitting on the floor had gone right up his rectum. I had envisioned a full-sized bottle of Prell, but he said it was only about a four-inch sample bottle. Louise took him back to one of the private rooms and positioned him on his side, staying there to comfort and stabilize him in that position. We both knew how that bottle had gotten up there and were kind enough not to ask any more questions. I anesthetized the rectal area as best I could and then inserted a vaginal speculum to maintain some dilation. I could then see the bottle enough to grab it with a tenaculum, rotate it longitudinally, and then deliver the bottle. It was still mostly full of shampoo and he did want it back. Sometime during the procedure, the patient said, "Oh, I'm so embarrassed."

"Think nothing of it," I said, "it happens every day." At this, Louise almost lost it. She was trying so hard not to laugh, and I thought she was going to drop him off the table. Louise loved a joke, and she got to see plenty of them because of her years of night work.

On another occasion, Louise and I were coming on for the night shift. We were told there was a suicidal man in his twenties being held in the cardiac room awaiting admission. He had been seen by the prior shift but was left unattended in the room during report, although there was a window into the room from where we were. During our report we heard a loud noise from that room, and we looked up to see that the man had properly applied the defibrillator paddles to his chest in an attempt to kill himself again. He was unsuccessful, but we were amazed that he could figure out how to use the defibrillator. The doctor who had seen the patient was known for not having much sympathy for suicidal patients. Louise asked this doctor what he wanted her to put on those paddle burns before the patient was taken upstairs. Without missing a beat, the doctor (whom I won't name) said "electrolyte jelly." This is the jelly applied to the skin so that the electric shock would flow better from the paddles and into the patient. Louise, wisely, did not follow that order.

About 2:00 a.m. on another morning, a tall, thin, scruffy, very agitated man walked in with some arterial bleeding from a knife wound to his arm. We could see on first glance that this was not a nice person, and he was probably high on drugs. He was led to the trauma room where he continued to act out in an uncooperative manner. He purposely flailed his injured arm about, spraying everything within range with blood. We requested multiple times that he recline on the bed so we could begin to care for him, but he continued to move about the room contaminating everything with his blood, which would have a high probability of carrying AIDS and/or hepatitis. Louise and I were the only ones there and we elected not to try to restrain him. There would have been two or three security guards somewhere in the building, but they were older and unarmed. The patient's purposeful motions made me think he was enjoying making the mess as a way of expressing himself. I tried again to talk him down and finally told him to cooperate or leave, which, to our surprise, he promptly did—all the while stating loudly that I would hear from his attorney in the morning. Our other options would have been to restrain and treat him against his will, for which we could be sued, or to wait until he passed out from blood loss and then we could treat him legally as an emergency. I don't know how many times I heard that exact same lawyer threat in my twenty-eight years in ERs, but I never did hear from any of their attorneys. Louise, again, wisely called the police to inform them of his leaving.

Later that night I spent about two hours suturing a friend of this patient, probably cut in the same fight. About a half hour later, I took a paramedic patch. They had picked up the patient who had left, and he requested that he not be transported back to St. Luke's. A short time later, a paramedic from that group came in to berate me, privately, for not treating that man the first time he came in. The city paramedics are given only one call at a time and won't get another until they place themselves back in service. At least three vehicles respond to each call—the initial fire truck that was closest, the paramedic truck, and usually an ambulance—and frequently a police car as well. Consequently, there are eight or more big men to accomplish their job, and if they need more, they call in more units. Contrast this with one nurse and one scrawny doctor trying to do their jobs in the ER. The Phoenix fire department encompasses the paramedic system and the ambulance transporters all under that tax-supported department. Have you ever looked at their equipment? They usually get everything they want or need. The Phoenix department, as I understood, had full-time public relations people to make sure that public opinion stayed high—and that tax money kept coming in. Of course, they are needed and do a good job, but I was a little jealous at their public-relations success, their equipment, and their option to call in more help when needed. St Luke's ER physicians have been deeply involved in paramedic training since they started in the 1980s. We helped them in doing many of the procedures that ER doctors would usually do, so that the important treatments could be started even before the patient arrived in the ER. The paramedics are gaining more autonomy now, but we physicians are still responsible for their actions, especially when we patch with them from a scene. Despite the above observations, I have the greatest respect for our paramedics. They work under some very difficult circumstances at times. As part of their training and ours, we spent time riding with them on their calls. I enjoyed their fire stations, their HBO TV, the meals they themselves would fix, the basketball games behind the stations, and the general camaraderie. I was amazed at how professional they were and how good they could be even to people who were obviously taking advantage of their services.

The late Dr. Michael Vance was a brilliant and dedicated St. Luke's ER physician and toxicologist who did much of the early paramedic training. He had a big hand in molding their program. I am told that he introduced himself on his very first day of work at St. Luke's by riding through the double doors into the ER on his motorcycle. Dr. John Gallagher took over after Dr. Vance. John has accompanied the Phoenix Fire Department on deployments such as the aftermath of 9-11 and Hurricane Katrina in 2005.

St. Luke's had three ER physicians who were also board certified in toxicology. They were the late Dr. Vance, the late Dr. Kunkel, and Dr. Ryan. They also had several fellows who went through their program. This was a very strong department and accounted for a good many admissions to the hospital. They started a poison control center with twenty-four-hour nurse phone service, backed up by the doctors. The toxicology service accounted for a good number of interesting stories.

Two boys were brought in from the desert one day who had been using peyote. The experience caused them to remove all their clothes and run around naked in the desert. They had champion sunburns and multiple cactus spines embedded in various places, but they didn't even notice. I guess some of the Indians use peyote in their religious services, but they never seem to get into trouble with it as these boys did. They were bouncing off the walls in the ER and got themselves admitted. I would guess that the nurses upstairs hated us for these admits.

Rattlesnake bites were always interesting, and each had a story. Many of the patients were playing with a snake while they were drunk, so it was easy to think that they deserved the bite. In one instance a man was trying to kiss his pet rattler when it bit him in the tongue. His tongue swelled rapidly and threatened to shut off his airway, so he got intubated immediately and was given lots of antivenin. The tube had to stay in several days until the tongue swelling receded.

A long-haul trucker appeared one day with a mean-looking bite to his index finger. He explained that he was trying to catch his rattlesnake to put it back in its glass jar. He explained that the truckers need to have something in the cab to keep "the natives" out when the trucker had to be away from the cab. He used to keep a dog in the cab, but worrying about feeding and potty breaks for the animal became too much trouble. He indicated that an increasing number of truckers were going to release snakes in their cabs and that it prevented more break-ins than a dog would. He said it had been quite effective in New York. He always put up a sign stating "Rattlesnake on Board" when he left the truck. When he came back, he just had to catch the snake and put it back in its jar. Having to catch the reptile each time would be bad enough, but I'd worry a lot about having an accident and being pinned in that truck with a broken jar and a loose snake.

One young man came in who had heard that oleander was poisonous. He wanted to kill himself, so he made malt out of oleander leaves and drank it. He only managed to make himself very sick and miserable, as gastrointestinal upset is the main poisonous effect of that plant.

Dr. Curry was one of those toxicology fellows who spent two or three years learning the specialty under the three toxicologists mentioned above. Dr. Kunkel was head of the program, and on Dr. Curry's very first day, he had admitted a critically ill rattlesnake bite to the ICU. Now, as it turned out, Dr. Curry had a great sense of humor that was a little off center sometimes. I was on duty, in-house that day and was in the patient's ICU room when Drs. Kunkel and Curry came in to evaluate the patient. Dr. Curry was at the patient's head and Dr. Kunkel was standing beside the bed. The lady was almost unconscious, but she said, "I have to poop." Remember that this was Dr. Curry's very first day and he was with the Big Chief of his service. Dr. Curry leaned closer to her and said, "Go ahead, Dr. Kunkel is there." The poor lady was only in her 40s, and she eventually died from complications of the bite. She did not deserve this accident. She had been riding her horse when the snake scared the animal. She was thrown off and the snake bit her. She received care for several days at a small hospital in Arizona and was flown to us when she was not improving. This is the only death I have ever seen from a rattlesnake bite, and it is, indeed, rare that the bites result in death. The large amounts of antivenin that are used for significant bites can be quite dangerous. Antivenin is actually horse serum containing high amounts of antibodies to rattlesnakes. Don't make me tell you how the horse gets these high antibodies. There is a danger of immediate anaphylaxis from the horse serum, and most patients get miserable serum sickness within a week.

One of our own favorite clerks came in one night. She had overdosed in a suicide attempt. She was nearly unconscious, and I had to intubate her. She had a stormy course, but she recovered fully and remains one of my favorite people. She always made sure that there was a cake on my birthdays and on one such occasion, she gave me a large teddy bear. Twyla always made up three large plates of her special cookies or candy on all the holidays, and I believe this human touch helped the fellow workers feel better toward me. I'd guess that the quality of those treats was something many had not often experienced.

Part of the hospital property faced Van Buren Street. That was unequivocally *the* address for prostitution, and we were right in the center of that area. The "hos" have apparently learned that if they have control of a man's clothes, they have control of him. I believe some of them hid or locked up the man's clothing as a condition for "the act" and for payment negotiations. Anyway, on several occasions, we had men appear in the ER with not a stitch on, telling a story that one could not believe. On one occasion Dr. Vance and Dr. Jackson (an attractive female cardiologist who worked in our ER) saw one of these unfortunate souls come into the building from a side door with *only* a hat on. They just looked at each other and didn't know what to say until Dr. Vance finally said, "Nice hat." We always sent these unfortunate naked men out wearing a pair of our scrubs.

The best way for me to get to work was to turn off the freeway at Washington Street and come up to St. Luke's from the south across that Van Buren Street. I wish I had a video of the young man blocking my way at seven o'clock one morning. He was gyrating/slithering down the middle of Nineteenth Street in nothing but a diaper draped across his chest just like the pictures we see of the typical New Year's baby. It looked like he was having a good experience with his drugs.

There was no light at Van Buren, and it was sometimes difficult to cross. Prostitutes always worked that corner, and they usually didn't bother me. They learn what the look is that could lead to money, and I didn't have it, as I was usually almost late for work by that time. One day, however, one of them came up to my magic floating Honda and rubbed her crotch on my closed driver's window. She left a smear on the window that certainly didn't attract me, and I couldn't wait to get it washed off.

Chris, a clerk in our ER, was a very nice looking trim black lady in her late fifties. We got off our shifts at the same time one day. Chris had dressed in all black that day and looked nice. I had gone out the far driveway and was driving along the street beside the hospital when I saw Chris, out of the corner of my eye, walking on the sidewalk in her all-black outfit. Wanting to talk with her about something, I pulled over to the curb near where she was. She had her hand on the door handle before I realized it was not Chris, but a local prostitute. I roared off (as much as that Honda could roar) and only hoped that no one had seen me almost pick up a prostitute. Maybe our daughter Kim was right to want me to retire before I got into trouble.

A local pimp brought one of his girls in one evening asking that we check her vagina for money. He said that she hid a fifty in there that was his. She agreed to the exam, or we couldn't have done it. I did the usual speculum and bimanual exam, and there was not a red cent in there. Our nurses talked at length with her, trying to get her some help and to get away out the back door, but she wanted to stay with him— I'm sure she feared for her life. We always give written discharge instructions upon dismissal. The nurse asked me what to write and I said, "to watch for any change," but she wouldn't do it. Police were there, but they couldn't do anything to help the girl either. One of them had worked in San Francisco and related that the pimps there would punish their girls by shoving a fish head first into the vagina.

Because of the direction of the gills, the fish would be very hard to remove.

You have probably heard the stories about how the illegal aliens plan their deliveries so as to be in the United States. The child is then a US citizen and, consequently, it is difficult to send the parents back to their countries of origin, which is most often Mexico. It would seem to me that this automatic citizenship could be changed with the proper legislation and the stroke of a pen, but it hasn't been. The hospitals near the Mexican border have literally hundreds of these deliveries each year and have for many years. We don't see a lot of that here in Phoenix, but occasionally they make it this far. I was called to the carport one day for such a delivery in progress. The baby had already been born and was on the floor of the front seat, in no distress. The father spoke some English, which was unusual, so I asked him what time the baby was born. Well, he said, it hit the floorboard about nine o'clock.

ER nurses don't like deliveries of any kind in their area and will do anything to facilitate moving the mother in labor somewhere else. There was no OB or pediatrics at St. Luke's, so we had nowhere to send them. We'd have to beg another hospital to take them. We didn't have to keep them (and shouldn't) because we didn't have those facilities. Anywhere else they might go, the receiving hospital must know it would probably be a no-pay situation. The hospitals have figured out how to get the state or federal government to pay some of those charges, which means that you and I pay.

One night in my first several years at St. Luke's, we received a drive-up—a man who had been shot multiple times. We had voluntary call lists with no teeth in them at that time, and I called seven different surgeons in an attempt to get him admitted and into surgery. My frustration level was very high at having a critical patient for whom we had no answers. We were spending time making calls (we had to talk with each of those surgeons and wait for each one to call back) while trying to stabilize the patient. I then started trying to find a trauma center to take the patient and to arrange transport. Maricopa County did agree to accept the patient, so I called the fire department paramedics to transport. They are not meant to do transports between hospitals, but this patient was too critical to be sent over in a private ambulance. I received some flak for that, but no one could tell me of a better plan.

I was always surprised that we could get *any* of the specialists to admit or promise to see patients referred from the ER. The pay from those cases has to be very low, and they are not really the type of folks one wants sitting in their office. The collection rate for ER work is often less than 50 percent. That directly affects the ER doctor's income, and one can only approach a reasonable income by working harder and seeing more patients. Those losses are also passed along to the bills that you and I receive when we have to be seen in an ER.

In the middle of another night, I was called to the area between our outer doors and the inside swinging doors where a fourteen-year-old was laying on the floor with a single gunshot wound to the chest. There was no one else in sight, so we had to discover the wound, move him into our trauma room, and begin treatment. The x-ray showed that his left chest was filled with blood, so he probably was shot through the heart. He died on our table. If he had walked into one of the five trauma centers, he would have had more rapid diagnosis and treatment and possibly had his chest opened in an attempt to repair the hole in the heart, but he would probably still have died. It was a while before his two brothers drove to our front door. They explained that after he was shot, they drove through our canopy five times but could not stop to let the patient out as the shooter's car was still chasing and shooting at them. On the fifth try, they rolled him out onto our driveway, and he must have been able to crawl to inside the outer door. Another strange aspect of this case was that when the mother arrived, she would not accept the fact that her son was indeed dead. I explained the facts to her many times and even showed her the body. She was ready to leave, and we thought she understood, but her final question was, "When will he be dismissed?" The police said that the eighteen-year-old brother driving the car was the actual target and the fourteen-year-old was hit by accident.

A man in his thirties signed in one night stating that he was going to die, and he did die about three hours later. He was alert and oriented with a low-grade fever and questionable stiffness to the neck. I was thinking meningitis and planned to do a spinal puncture for diagnosis. When possible, one should get a head CT before a spinal tap to rule out a bleed or other pressure lesion in the head. If that is present, removal of spinal fluid may cause the brain to herniate down through the foramen magnum resulting in probable death. The man went to CT, but when he came back, he was seizing. I had to intubate him and treat the seizures. Fortunately, this time, a neurologist was in the building who accepted the patient in admission. He did accomplish the tap and said that the spinal fluid was purulent (infected) and that the man would soon die, which he did. He had meningococcal meningitis, which is the rapidly fatal kind. All of us who had been exposed to him received injectable and oral prophylactic antibiotics.

There were some cases not so serious. A teenage girl came in during the day with both legs blue. She had a brand-new pair of jeans, and her "cyanosis" was the color rubbing off on her legs.

We did an unsuccessful code on a two-year-old one day who was killed by a bookcase that fell on him. Maybe that is why I am so insistent that all of the heavy pieces in our daughters' homes be secured to the wall or floor.

I was knocked totally unconscious by a young man on PCP one day. He was reclining on a cart and we were mildly restraining him so that he would not hurt himself or others. A nurse (not Louise) was holding his right arm and I had the left. He suddenly came across with his right fist, striking me solidly on the chin. The last I remember is that my legs wouldn't hold me up and I went down. His left fist, then loose, bloodied the nurse's nose on the right. I don't believe I was out for long, as when I awakened, a huge pile of people had covered the patient on the floor. I added myself to that pile but couldn't really make my arms do anything. I told Twyla the story when I got home at the end of my shift and she very seriously said, "Well, what did you do to aggravate him?"

There had been extensive news coverage of Andre Agassi playing in a tennis tournament in Australia. The news also reported that he would be headed for Phoenix in his private jet, probably for more tennis. That evening, we received a call from the Agassi plane indicating that they had a man on board seriously ill with seizures and that two doctors on the plane had already given him IV Valium. St. Luke's was close to the airport (Sky Harbor) and received most of the in-flight emergency patients. We fully expected an ambulance with lights and sirens. Soon, a man walked in and sat in a chair in admissions, stating that he was that person from the Agassi plane. He got checked in and moved to a room where he had another "seizure." It didn't look too real, but I think he got some Valium IV anyway. When he had the next seizure, I told him to just stop it, which he did. I told him that I was onto his scam and he should move on. Meanwhile, the clerk called the airport and found that Andre Agassi's plane had not yet landed. I then felt much more comfortable calling his bluff. He stayed around, though, still insisting that he needed anti-seizure medication. We asked him how he had arrived, and he said the limousine had dropped him at the door. I asked him to call them to come get him and to let me see the limousine when it arrived. This guy knew we didn't believe anything he was saying, but he persisted, as if he himself believed it. He made his call for transportation and, much to my surprise, called me to the door when his transportation arrived. I found him talking to a taxi driver—but the driver was in a sports jacket. The patient kept trying to convince me that the standard taxi sitting in our drive was a limousine, even as we both stood looking at it. I asked the driver if he had maybe been driving a limousine earlier or had seen this patient before. Sure, he said, earlier this evening, when he brought him here from Good Sam ER in his taxi. The taxi driver, I could tell, was getting a little uneasy transporting this guy, given the above questions. The patient, however, eased the driver's fears by handing him four crisp new one-hundred-dollar bills. I heard the driver say, "I'll take you anywhere you want."

There are people who are "professional patients" and make their livings or get their kicks that way. There are two types. The first is the drug addict and/or dealer who is especially good at manipulation. They charm or threaten doctors to get their drugs and cause tremendous disruption to emergency departments, but they make a very good living off what they get and sell. Percocet has been worth about fifty dollars per pill on the street.

The second group is the type who seem to get their kicks from manipulation and from seeing just how far they can go with their little games. These aren't always centered around narcotics, and I'm not sure how they make their living. These individuals are skilled at carrying a scenario to ridiculous extremes, almost as if the people around them are hypnotized. They must use these skills outside the ER to make a good dishonest living. There is likely a psychiatric diagnosis for this second group. I almost feel sorry for them.

The next patient was likely a combination of both types. He flew into Phoenix on a commercial airline. He was so smooth and personable that he convinced those around him that he was a professional football player. He carried this deception so far that stewardesses from his plane brought him roses during his hospitalization. His presentation in the ER was that of being in a sickle cell crisis, which is extremely painful and hard to disprove. He got me to give him 800 mg of Demerol IV during his ER stay, which is a far larger total than I had ever given anyone. He continued to complain of pain and did not improve, so I was able to talk a doctor into admitting him. The admitting doctor would have consults available with addiction specialists, toxicologists, and psychiatrists. It was determined that he was totally feigning his pain and symptoms, but it still took three days to get him out of the hospital. This person will not get better but will spend his entire life fooling doctors and others until he overdoses one day.

Even relatively normal people can be difficult at times, especially now with the wait time occasionally stretching out to eight hours. The anger was almost palpable on those nights, and the first part of the visit would be spent trying to win the patient and family back over and that sometimes didn't happen. We weren't allowed to park our own cars very close to the door, and I remember being uncomfortable and hyper alert in walking to my car, especially during the night shift changes. One such night at St. Luke's I was heading to the car when some car lights came up behind me and there was a click that sounded just like a shotgun being pumped. I hit the dirt (or cement, as it was) and then realized that the noise was only car tires passing over the entrance grate into the parking area directly behind me. The people in that car must have wondered what happened to that old man in their lights, but they didn't stop to ask.

Most of the deviant behavior that I've mentioned comes to these people naturally, almost as a gift. There are so many resources available, though, even for normal people to learn how to get what they want or how to disrupt lives. There are businesses that masquerade as supply centers for law enforcement personnel or homeowners wanting protection. It is, however, the first place I would go if I were a burglar, or if I wanted supplies for a variety of criminal activities. They have entire books on topics such as how to get even with your doctor, neighbor, and parents, for example. These books teach all manner of dirty tricks that will cause major and serious disruption to the lives of their targets. They also tell how to kill without being caught, even going into how to dispose of the body. The wand or club that was used on figure skater Nancy Kerrigan's legs was purchased at one of these supply shops.

I thought that I had just about finished the St. Luke's stories when I quit writing at midnight last night. More stories kept coming through the night, however, and by this morning I had seven Post-it pads filled with ideas about other stories. I hope that getting this all written will act as a cathartic and stop the bad dreams that I have been having nightly since retirement. You might wonder why *anyone* would want to do this work, and I have asked that many times myself. As time went on, all of the risks increased greatly. There was a risk of physical injury both from the patients and from the disruption of sleep patterns from doing shift work. The exposure to serious or fatal illnesses increased greatly in later years, mostly due to AIDS and hepatitis. The malpractice risk-to-benefit ratio became so unfavorable that it seemed almost foolish to continue working. We had accumulated assets by that time, all of which were at risk each shift I worked. Malpractice insurance covered us only to one million dollars per case, with a three-million-dollar lifetime limit. It is not hard for awards to go over that, and after that, personal assets are taken. Walking up to that door for a shift became more difficult as time went on. The ER doctor is likely to be named in suits against other doctors in the community, because we are seeing their sickest patients and those at higher risk. The office doctors are also not above placing blame upon the ER physician and some even take the patient's side in the case. I do realize, however, that many others perform dirty, risky, unpleasant jobs (nurses, teachers, and sewer cleaners) and these do the work without the financial rewards.

ER technicians are trained on the job to do much of the work that nurses used to do, and most get very good at their jobs. Many are frustrated wannabe nurses or doctors. We had a very good male tech at St. Luke's who told a story about a time that he was moving his piano with help from friends. Since it wasn't far, he decided to move it during the night, when he could just roll it down McDowell Street to his next apartment. The cops came by, of course, and thought that he might be stealing the piano. He told them it was his. They consulted for a moment and then told him he'd better be able to play that piano, so he gave them a concert in the middle of McDowell Street.

The same tech told of an orthopod (orthopedic doctor) with an especially unpleasant demeanor who was very difficult to work with. The orthopod was applying a full-body cast to a patient reclining on an ortho table, and the tech tried twice to tell him that he was encasing part of the table within the cast. This doctor essentially would not let the tech finish his comments, so the tech helped him finish the cast and let the truth be known when it came time to move the patient. The cast had to be taken off and reapplied.

The same tech bought himself a new used Cadillac while working with us. He was so proud of it and couldn't quit talking about the car. To protect his valuable investment, he parked it in the area reserved for patient parking, close to the ER door, then went out to look at it several times each shift. I thought it would be funny to apply the fake scratch patch to his rear fender, but I don't believe he thought it was all that funny.

Dr. Curry liked to call the ER clerks and just make animal noises. Remodeling of the ER had been completed and an opening date for its first use was chosen. Only when the girls sat at their desks for the first time did anyone realize that no phone lines had been installed. It was funny that there was a functioning TTY phone for the deaf. It was designed so that messages would be typed back and forth between the deaf person and the recipient. I'm sure that it was a federal mandate that it be installed. It was in such a prominent place, taking up valuable desk space, that I'll bet its location was also mandated by the legislation. None of us liked that phone, and in twelve years we never received a call from a real deaf person. We did receive frequent wrong number calls though, and a favorite response to those, after the line was clear, was to yell loudly into the phone, "SPEAK UP!"

In the department it was known that I untied all bows. Sue was a nice, short, somewhat-proper nurse. As usual, I was dressed in scrubs, and it was shift-change time in the central area. Sue decided that it would be a funny time to get even with me for something by untying the bow in the front of my scrub pants. I, of course, made no effort to stop that pair of pants from falling to the floor and may even have subtly helped the process along. Sue knew then that the pants were on the way to my ankles. Sue got red as a beet and was so flustered that she was making uncoordinated motions with her hands and arms until she finally decided that she had to tie that bow again. All ended well and I wasn't exposed, but she never repeated the act.

The waiting room for our department was not very big. It was like a wide hallway along the north wall just beside the outside double doors. The windows to the outside were uncovered, which made one feel very exposed when in that room. In an attempt to make the area a little more pleasant, a TV was hung on the wall and a coffee maker installed. Those conveniences lasted only a few days before they were stolen. The security guards saw them being carried into one of the apartments in The Projects, directly across the street. The Projects were one-story government housing for the poor, and they surrounded the hospital on two sides. Our security was not allowed to retrieve the property.

There were several instances of ER doctors using narcotics that I know of. These doctors always wanted to give narcotic injections to their own patients, which should have seemed a little strange. They would draw up the narcotic and pocket that loaded syringe. They would then have a previously prepared syringe in another pocket filled with saline and would give that to the patient. At times when they could obtain access to a vial of narcotic, they would withdraw some and again place it into their pocket, then use the other syringe of saline to replenish the vial with the same amount—so that counts and amounts would still be correct. These were good, caring physicians who would not want to hurt patients, yet their addiction was stronger. One was a good family man, but he overdosed and died. I had worked with him at several ERs and would have trusted him with my life.

I transported my personal items and billfold to St. Luke's in a scuffed-up leather briefcase. I would park the case on the vanity in the ER doctor's bathroom and would seem to need a toothbrush or something out of it quite often during the twelve- to-twenty-four-hour shifts. Twyla made sure I always had one or two twenty-dollar bills in my billfold. I thought I was losing my mind because there often seemed to be one less than I remembered. It turned out that the cleaning man had been taking a twenty-dollar tip on the days I was there. He never took all the money, and he must have counted on his victims not missing the amount taken. Our security caught him with a tiny security camera, which was pretty high tech for that time. One day, that scrubby case got a leather polish and shine and looked brand new. No one would admit to doing that, but I suspect either Dr. Ryan or Dr. Fisher.

Drs. Ryan and Fisher both have roots in Iowa; Dr. Ryan in College Springs and Grinnell and Simpson College, and Dr. Fisher had relatives in Yorktown. We met Dr. Fisher's family at Luke AFB where we were both flight surgeons. Our service overlapped for over a year. He was already at St. Luke's when I arrived. We did some barroom genealogy once and found that he was distantly related to both Twyla and me—way back.

There was a tall, dark, and handsome ENT specialist based in the St. Luke's office building, which was a new wing attached to the hospital. He appeared very successful at treating migraines with lidocaine injections around various branches of the cranial nerves. He did lots of injections into the area of the supraorbital nerves and was starting to have us do that for him on his patients. I believe he had published some articles on this treatment. This idea may have been a little controversial, but I believe there are some parallel successes that used the same reasoning; that is, if the pain or spasm can be totally relieved for a short time it will go away, or the spasm will relax. This is the basis for the new "muscle energy" method of manipulation where the muscle in spasm is held for about ninety seconds in a shortened position until it stays relaxed. There are also those who are very enthusiastic about treating fibromyalgia with lidocaine injections into the tender trigger areas. One more is the idea of using adequate narcotic dosages, saying that long-term pain may actually be aborted by these doses. Anyway, I digress. Dr. Fisher was on duty in-house this day, and he was called to the ENT doctor's office where he found that the doctor had put a gun in his mouth and fired. There was nothing to do. This was such a waste and such a shock to those of us who had worked with him.

St. Luke's Hospital was designed with eight floors and a nice, small patio outside each room. As you might guess, there were suicide jumps off those upper patios, so the doors out had to be bolted and the patios not used. I was never on one of those patios in my entire sixteen years there.

A psychiatric patient was brought over from the psych wing to be evaluated—after he had tried to kill himself by jumping off the dresser in his room onto his head. He was holding his neck a little stiffly, but an injury didn't seem too likely with that history alone. He was waiting on his cart for an x-ray and wanted me to blow his nose for him. I placed a tissue box on his chest and told him to blow his own nose. The film showed, however, that he had an unstable fracture of the odontoid process of his C2 vertebra, the vertebral process that our heads turn on. He was firmly packaged, then admitted until morning when he received a halo vest to stabilize his head and neck. After this, I suspect that we blew his nose for him whenever he wanted. He did okay with his neck. I don't know what they were able to do about his jumping problem.

When an x-ray is taken, there is a medium-pitched beep that lasts about one second at the exact time of exposure. All in the area are to have protected themselves from the exposure to that ray. We had one x-ray tech who could exactly duplicate that sound with his vocal cords. He would drive people crazy by giving that "beep" at the most inopportune times when lots of folks were in the x-ray room and unprotected. I have tried very hard to learn to do that, but just can't get the sound to be believable.

I lost an in-house post tracheotomy patient once. He had cancer of the vocal cords but looked strong and healthy in his '60s. The trach was done to bypass the cancer and allow him to get air into his lungs. A known complication of tracheotomies is that the lower edge of the tube can erode a large vessel inside the trachea where it lies, and the blood runs down into the lungs. I knew what had to be done, which was to remove the trach tube and insert into the same hole an endotracheal tube and blow up the balloon. That would keep the blood from running into the lungs and still allow air passage through that tube until the surgeon could fix the bleeder. The patient was naturally agitated and was thrashing and spitting so much blood that I could not physically get and keep that tube in place. This one has bothered me, and I wonder whether someone else could have accomplished it or whether I should have asked for help earlier. The tube went in easily once he was quiet, but it was too late by then.

The colon is about the last five feet of the bowel and terminates at the rectum. A gregarious young man was seen for abdominal pain, which proved to be a ruptured colon. The diagnosis would have been difficult to make, except for the history, which he willingly gave. His lover had been "fisting" him. He had to explain that to me. It apparently involves the lover inserting his entire fist through the rectum and into the lower colon, then making whatever movements would cause the desired sexual stimulation. Now, most of us who lack tolerance and understanding would be somewhat upset if someone did that to us, but apparently it is a source of great pleasure for the initiated few. This man was very philosophical about the whole stream of events, though. I distinctly remember him saying, as he was rolling down the hall to surgery, "If you play, you have to pay."

Gerbilling is a word that I cannot find in Webster's. It must be a street word for an activity somewhat similar to that in the above paragraph. I have not personally seen any patient injured by gerbilling, but it is a common ER story. Gerbil cages have plastic tubing in which the rodent runs incessantly. The "gerbillee" probably with the help of a "gerbillor" inserts one end of the tubing into the rectum. They then scare the poor animal so that it runs out the end of the tube and into the colon of the patient. The terminal movements and scratching of the rodent must then provide the sexual high that is sought. I have no knowledge of what happens next, but I surmise that a fair number of these would need ER care at some point. Here is a great chance to start another support group. I did find the word gerbilling in Wikipedia. They claim that the whole thing is an urban legend and that there is no medical confirmation of such activity, so it's probably best to forget this paragraph.

George was one of my favorite gay nurses, an unabashed flaming homosexual. He had a great sense of humor which often involved making fun of himself. I once asked him to insert a CO2 suppository into a patient's rectum. It was a new type that released the CO2 gas into the bowel and caused movement in that way, made by the Beutlich Company in Germany. George soon came out of the room just rolling in laughter. He showed me the label and said "Do you know who makes this suppository? It's the butt-lick company."

Our ER department traditionally had a Christmas party in which "white elephant" gifts were exchanged. We would all save our most obnoxious, non-usable items throughout the year to place into the exchange, and some of the worst items would be given again year after year. George opened the gift that he had drawn one year, and it was a pair of beautiful pink glass slippers. I'm not sure that it wasn't a setup, maybe even by George himself. Anyway, George produced lots of laughs by the various ways that he showed his extreme appreciation for the gift.

Since my teen years, hypnosis has been an interest of mine. I used it somewhat on stage as part of the family magic shows, for deliveries in general practice, and for reduction of dislocated shoulders in the ER. Hypnosis is especially good for muscle relaxation, which is what is mostly needed to reduce a shoulder. I used it with success about six times and once even through an interpreter. It never failed. The nurses loved it because they could just put me in a room with the patient and in about a half hour, they could apply the sling and the patient could go home. The standard treatment otherwise was IVs with drugs for conscious sedation and then a long period of observation for the wake-up period. This would tie up several of the nursing staff for a considerable time and entailed more risk for the patient.

A certain percentage of the disabled go to the ERs because it is easier for them to obtain access and get help. One can't blame them—they have to do what they have to do to survive and get care—but this does put an extra burden on the ER because these people require more help and time. Many are obese, partly because of their inability to exercise. A small percentage have learned to use their disability to get what they want and when they want it. One can see that the ER gets a larger percentage of really difficult patients, including the disabled, severe traumas, those too messy to be seen in offices, the emotionally unstable, and addicts. All this goes on while at the same time needing to see many who don't need to be there. Most disabled do understand and appreciate that they need more help to manipulate their wheelchairs in public, but a few will say "excuse me" in a demanding way and *expect* everyone to get out of their way or help them. I guess we should be glad it is not us needing the help. If you have triplets, don't get a three-across stroller.

Twyla had her hysterectomy and substernal thyroid surgeries, and I had a transurethral resection (TUR) while at St. Luke's, under their insurance. We could not have been treated better. We didn't even know then what it meant to pay anything extra for medical care. It was a different time. Twyla's substernal thyroid surgery was especially stressful. She'd had a tracheal deviation on her chest x-rays for some time, but one of the radiologists at St. Luke's suggested she get a CAT scan of her chest. This showed a fist-sized mass above her heart, intermixed with her major vessels. The differentials for this mass were almost all bad. She went to surgery and the mass was removed intact by Dr. Goldberg. Pathology reported the mass was benign thyroid tissue. He had to extend the incision up her left throat in order to tie off the vessels to the lesion so that it could be removed. I seem to remember that Twyla's father Mervil had surgery for a substernal thyroid.

I had a frightening experience during this time period in which I developed extensive lymphatic streaking up the left arm into the axilla with large tender lymph nodes. There were multiple distinct streaks with much axillary tenderness. I started high-dose antibiotics, which, in my experience, had always cured this "blood poisoning." This condition went on for about six weeks during which time I saw three different physicians, and none could tell me a diagnosis or why it was not responding to usual therapy. An infectious disease specialist wanted me to stop treatment and to go without any medicine for ten days and then come back for cultures. I expected more from him. I did not miss any work with this but was uncomfortable and very worried. It eventually got better, no thanks to anyone. My reading since then has suggested that this was sporotrichosis, a fungal infection from skin punctures from plants It could have been treated with antifungals. I was doing extensive work at that time with thorny plants at the Cholla house and, I'm sure, had a puncture to the dorsum or my left hand from pyracantha or bougainvillea.

Payson is a mountain town of ten thousand. It sits at approximately 7000' elevation and thinks it is a rough old-time mountain cowboy town. They even have log-rolling contests and rodeos each year. St. Luke's staffed their ER for several years with our ER doctors. At any rate, we insisted upon being full voting members of their staff, which made the local doctors uncomfortable—and I don't blame them. Because of the distance and the fact that the volume was not great, we worked twenty-four-hour shifts—so that there was a replacement doctor driving up the mountain at seven o'clock each morning. I did enjoy having breakfast at one of the Payson restaurants every morning when headed for home. The people in town weren't so tough, but there were some real mountain men out in the hills.

One of these mountain men came in one day with a severe scalp laceration. He had fallen off his mule way up in the mountains and had hit his head on a rock. I asked him how he had stemmed the bleeding, and he said that he just put his old hat back on "real tight" and the mule took him home. Indeed, he did have an old felt hat with him, which had obviously been part of him for some time, and it was caked with blood. I sutured the extensive laceration and instructed him to keep it clean. He promised to do that, but as he was leaving, we noted he put that dirty old hat firmly back on his head, right over the exposed sutures.

Because of the elevation, it was cooler in the summer in Payson than in the valley, and many came up to spend time away from the heat. An ASU professor came in one summer day with a severe allergic reaction to shrimp. My favorite local ER nurse was on that day, and she had an IV, adrenalin, Benadryl, and cortisone into him almost before I could order it. He recovered well and told us of his experience with his first allergic reaction at Scottsdale Memorial Hospital some time before. He had been to their ER and was treated for an upper respiratory infection with a prescription for penicillin. As he was walking out accompanied by the doctor, he saw a large room off to the side and near the front door. He asked, "What do you do in this room?" The doctor answered, "Oh that's where we put patients who we think aren't going to make it." You guessed it. He went out, took his first dose of penicillin, had a reaction, and was taken right back to Scottsdale Memorial where he awakened in *that* room.

We received a young man one night who had been driving, drunk and alone, and simply ran into a tree. His neck x-ray was okay, but we admitted him anyway, for some reason. The admitting surgeon ordered a CT of the neck the next morning because his neck was still sore. The CT showed a cervical spine fracture. We sent the patient to Phoenix, probably to St. Joseph Hospital. There was some talk of a suit over that, but it was not possible for me to have obtained a CT during the night, and I had no real reason to transfer him, as he had no neurological defects. Like one of the nurses said, his injury may have had *something* to do with the fact that he was drunk and ran into a tree.

We received a man one evening who had been shot squarely in the back of his head. He was in and out of consciousness and I assumed that he would die. When he came back from x-ray, however, the film showed that the bullet did not enter the cranium but coursed around the skull where it stopped in the soft tissues near the right temple. His symptoms would be a result of concussion, which had to be significant. We had called for a helicopter early, so we packaged him up and sent him to a trauma center in the valley. A standard joke in small town emergency departments is that if you receive anything more severe than a paper cut, you order a CBC and a helicopter. I know of no reason that he should not have done all right.

During all of this commotion, the sheriff's officers brought in a screaming "psych" patient. I could not get to her very quickly and heard that she kept referring to a grave, a rattlesnake, and a gun. When I finally got free, I was able to get the story from the officers. Her boyfriend, the one who was shot, had been very upset at her and was digging a grave. He had put a rattlesnake into it and was going to put this woman into that hole as punishment. He made the mistake of laying his revolver down while he dug. The woman wasn't going to submit to being shot and buried, so she picked up the gun and shot him in the back of the head. It took a while to quiet her down, but she'd had a stressful night. I don't know what happened to her, but I suspect she may have been punished by the legal system with only a slap to the wrist.

Another shooting in Payson was a young man brought in with five gunshot wounds—four in the chest and one in the neck. Looking at the projected path of any one of these wounds suggested that each alone should have been fatal. I assumed that he would also die in our ER, but I ordered the CBC and helicopter anyway. We did what we could and again shipped him off to a trauma center in the valley. Since he lived through that first hour, I assume he also made it. By this time, it seemed that no one died from bullet wounds in Payson. The story finally came to us that the woman who shot him was also his girlfriend. He was a bible-carrying schizophrenic and had been introducing himself to others that way. The girlfriend got very tired of all that religious talk, so she shot him—not once, but five times. When the paramedics arrived, she was running around his house looking for more bullets. An interesting sidebar to this case is that I had to go to Globe to testify in the case against the girlfriend. I completed my testimony and the court took a break. I went outdoors to relax on a cement bench with another young lady who was sitting out there alone and smoking. I asked her what she had to do with the case, and she said she was the girlfriend shooter. I think my good dress shoes got scuffed getting back into the courthouse.

We all looked forward to 7:00 a.m. when our shifts would be over and we would be relieved. One day, Jim Gross was scheduled to replace me, but he didn't come. About 8:00 a.m. we received an ambulance from the Beeline Highway. I knew it was Jim when he was pulled out feet first and I recognized his pointed, polished shoes. He seemed to be in pretty good shape. His chest x-ray showed a white area which turned out to be only a lung contusion, but I wasn't sure it was not the beginning of a larger bleed. He was helicoptered to St. Luke's, and I was relieved of my shift later that day. When Jim returned to work, he gave me pictures of his Honda, which was totally destroyed in this one-car accident. I believe he sent pictures to the Honda Motor Company, showing how his car had saved him. Several of his tires came off in the accident, and they were never found.

It seemed that I was always unsettled at St. Luke's and looking for greener grass. I took at least four part-time jobs that I thought might lead to full time work at other places. Some of them appeared to have higher income as well as harder work. I was also looking for variety so my skills in some areas could be maintained. The part-time jobs also provided some additional income, which we needed with four in schools. I never totally cut ties to St. Luke's until 1996, but I had about three "affairs" with various emergency departments and groups before then. Both Drs. Bursey and Ryan, as well as St. Luke's administration, were always very supportive and seemed genuinely interested in my forays.

John C. Lincoln Emergency Room (JCL ER) provided part-time work for me during much of the sixteen years at St. Luke's, and I was always treated well there. Both JCL and St. Luke's were good enough to work with me in meshing my schedules. JCL had their ER as well as three urgent care centers, which all provided me some variety in the types of work because of the different levels of severity that came into each facility. As a matter of fact, my last year of work was exclusively at JCL. I appreciated the ERs that provided the physicians enough help, such as techs who could set up for closing lacerations or apply casts and splints, often better than we could.

Another job outside of St. Luke's was with a group of three who had the contract to staff the Desert Valley ER at Fortieth Street and Bell. Three physicians were not enough to cover the ER 24-7, so I was hired full time with the idea of becoming a partner. The emergency department was unusually busy. One night, when evaluating the group's financial records, I found that the three partners, while at home, were *each* making considerably more than I did while *working* my shift. The timing and terms of joining as a partner remained vague. There should have been a buy-in, the amount increasing as accounts receivable grew. I had no business knowledge, and the partners were very business savvy. I finally realized that they had no reason to ever take me as a partner. I worked heavily part time at Desert Valley for about a year, but I had continued doing some shifts at John C. Lincoln and maintained full time hours at St. Luke's during that same time. I never had a shortage of part time work. I must have always felt a fear of being without work, as I had trouble turning down extra shifts when they were offered.

On one other occasion I worked full time at both Thunderbird Hospital ER and at St. Luke's for about a year but decided to not go exclusive with Thunderbird. It was around this time that the Thunderbird and St. Luke's groups were considering merging.

I did some part-time work with some of the other doctors from St. Luke's ER group for the Call Doc group out of Chicago. They had four vans operational in Chicago and then started one in Phoenix. Their stated purpose was to provide house-call service to patients on an interim basis—a service that was meant to benefit the patients as well as their physicians. I understood it was to be supplemental house-call care for patients who could not see a physician in the office for one reason or another. This was not a twenty-four-hour service, and there was no means for admission or long-term care. However, the service *was* being used as the only provider of care to many homebound and elderly patients without primary care physicians. We ended up providing the *only* care to some patients in the many group homes scattered across Phoenix. They had care from nine to five, when we could get there, and none after 5:00 p.m. or on weekends. The patients would have to be taken to emergency rooms when we weren't available. This was not my idea of good care, but the owners didn't seem to mind. There was a lot we didn't understand about this business. The owner and his administrative people, of which there were many, would fly in to meet with us and oversee the service, and they could talk only of expansion and advertising when we already had more business than we could do with one van. We would sometimes drive across the city for calls. They never considered adding another van or additional personnel, and they talked repeatedly about how much money they could spend on their high living. It seemed almost as if they were laundering someone's money. The office space was large and occupied what looked like a high-rent building. It was on the third floor—not easy for resupplying the van. We had an office Christmas party at our house that year. Two of the Chicago administrative people came, as well as the two office help/tech/van drivers. The girls were so drunk that they just giggled through the meal while the Chicagoans continued their talk about expansion of the business. Dr. Ryan and another of the St. Luke's ER doctors were in attendance also. We decided then that something was seriously wrong, and none of us worked for them anymore. We heard that the Chicago-Phoenix division of Call Doc ceased operations about four months later. I would sure like to know the whole story. The original Call Doc Company is still operating out of San Diego and has about a thousand physicians nationwide working for them, so I believe that the basic idea was good. The vans had been equipped with x-ray, limited rapid lab, and meds, and could do IVs. The x-ray quality was terrible, but we were able to diagnose bilateral hip fractures on one lady and get her admitted to St. Luke's for care.

A man and his girlfriend, both perhaps in their mid-fifties, showed a combination of nervousness and giddiness as they sat on the cart behind the curtain at JCL ER. Their wait had been long, so I expected more anger. When I asked what the problem was, they looked at each other sheepishly and giggled. I said, "I think there is a story here, let me get a chair." The lady had a huge hematoma under the tongue, with the frenulum torn from its base. Without any further coaxing, she volunteered that she had been giving her boyfriend oral sex and she said, "I zigged when I should have zagged." I referred them to an oral surgeon for follow-up and wrote down the discharge instructions discreetly to help protect their little secret.

The two trauma rooms at JCL were busy, sometimes seeing up to twelve traumas in a day. Meanwhile, other patients would continue to be seen in the other fifteen beds. One need only listen to the Phoenix area news to understand why we were so busy. When a trauma arrival was called over the hospital-wide intercom, a scurry of people showed up, each ready to do their part if needed. Blood is drawn, IVs inserted, tubes inserted as needed, diagnostic imaging is done in the room on the table, and blood is not far away. The trauma surgeon and anesthesiologist are part of the team, as well as one ER doctor. Many deaths occurred in those rooms, so we were always glad to see a good survival. Since I was mostly part time, I was not usually in the trauma room.

One patient came in and was assigned to someone else, but I watched as he was placed on the trauma room table. He was on his side due to a two-by-four piece of lumber that had pierced him through the abdomen, back to front. The patient had been a passenger in a convertible accident in which the car was thrown backward into a patio and the patient was pierced by the one of the two-by-four supports for the structure. The fire department had to cut the lumber off about two feet in front and two feet behind the patient in order to transport him. The patient went to surgery, where they found that the board had miraculously avoided all major structures. It was removed, and I heard that he did well. As an example of sick ER humor, some referred to this as the shish kebab case.

A dirty, street-like couple were in the isolation room because of multiple purulent, draining skin lesions. The diagnosis was fairly easy, since the worst of the lesions were in areas which could be reached for self-injection. They had used up all the veins that they could reach and were now "skin popping" their narcotics. They were injecting under the skin in any area, and these spots frequently became infected. I talked with them about their condition and why they were getting these infections, knowing it would likely do no good by the next day. As I was leaving the room, they asked if they could have sex. I thought for a moment and decided that since they both probably had the same bacteria, I said they could. I went back to my dictation area, dictated their charts, and wrote discharge instructions. The nurse then went back into the room to dismiss them and *they were having sex.* I hadn't meant sex right there and now, but to them, it was probably the best place they would find all night. Believe me, a story this good spreads rapidly to every ER in town.

As a follow-up to the above story, the very next night I was seeing a sweet young woman in that same room. She was newly married and had honeymoon cystitis, a bladder infection that can occur while the newlyweds are getting accustomed to each other's bacteria. It was an easy case, and as I was writing her prescription she said, "Now can we have sex?"

It couldn't be helped. I broke out into uncontrolled laughter. After recovering from my inappropriate behavior, I got to tell her the story from the night before. She understood and enjoyed the story—and I enjoyed telling it again.

An eighteen-year-old motorcyclist was brought in with injuries that proved fatal, and it fell to me to tell the mother who was waiting in the grieving room. It was a small, stuffy room, and I always hated giving bad news in such a tight area. One never knows what the recipient of the news will do. This mother was appropriate, but very grief-stricken. When she had recovered control, she said she was sorry to have made such a scene, but her other son had met the same fate about a year before and she received that news in this same room. She had more reason to hate that room than I did.

We all hated to do rape examinations. There were so many aspects to this examination process, and everything had to be done correctly, or the case could be lost in court. Many samples had to be taken in a precise way to be valid. We then would need to do what could be done to prevent pregnancy and treat prophylactically for the contagious diseases that could be treated, as well as treating any injuries. One would almost certainly receive a summons to testify a year later. At this time, a violent rapist was on the loose who had killed several girls. One evening one of his victims came in alive. He had left her for dead in a lonely desert area near Highway 17 north of town. She was able to walk to the highway where a trucker assisted her. She was barefoot and covered with cactus spines from walking through the desert in the dark. She had some injuries, one of which was a fracture of one of her small fingers with bone exposed, but none were life threatening. I testified on this case, and I believe the guy was put away. The lawyers are civil to us until they are done with our testimony, but none ever gave me any friendly follow-up on cases we'd spent hours on.

A very nice thirty-year-old arrived with severe lacerations over the proximal phalanx of several fingers of his right hand, and the injury involved tendons. He indicated he had sustained the cut while helping a friend move a glass tabletop. We talked about how dangerous those tops can be, and I was especially interested because we had one. I promised him that I would be very careful with that top from now on. Repair of flexor tendons of the hand has to be done by hand surgeons in a surgical setting. Our hand surgeon on call reluctantly agreed to see the patient the next day. I assured him that this was a "regular guy" and not the usual ER trash and that he would like this patient—as did the ER personnel. I closed the wounds loosely for the night, knowing that the sutures would be removed the next day for the deeper surgery. A beautiful Phoenix Police homicide officer waited to talk with me about this guy when I arrived for my next shift at JCL. The story was that he'd had a disagreement with a transvestite on Van Buren Street and had cut up that person with a machete, with a fatal outcome. The laceration apparently occurred when the patient had to grab onto the machete sometime during that murder. I had to testify on this case, too. Again, I don't know the outcome. The court seemed interested in what impression the patient had made on the ER personnel. I had to say that we all liked and trusted him. My estimate of the age of the wound did not agree with the timing of the crime, and I hoped that he did not get off because of that discrepancy.

Another circumstance that makes wild stories is where a person is injured by a tool or machine the continues to run when the individual is rendered suddenly unconscious by a medical condition—such as stroke or hypoglycemia. The tool (saw, vibrator, sander, etc.) continues to run and can do extensive damage while in contact with the person. The tool continues to do its damage until the person is discovered and the machine is unplugged from the wall or shut off. You can make up your own stories based upon this scenario. If the paramedics don't give us the whole story, we can miss what really happened. I don't want to bore you with more vibrator stories, but batteries are so much improved now that even if not plugged into the wall, much damage can be done. My family gets annoyed at me occasionally because I see danger in everything—but the truth is, I have seen everything. Batteries have to be stored or disposed of properly so that the positive and negative ends do not touch. It they spark, they could burn your house down with you in it. When with the family, I see circumstances daily that have injured or killed someone. I see much to worry about and still often do really stupid things myself. How can I expect others to know?

The twenty-year-old male who walked in one day was somewhat uncooperative and had a fracture of his left forearm. Certain conditions required us to get police clearance before he could be released. His story and injuries made no sense, and two huge policemen spent about thirty minutes interviewing him. They eventually determined that he could go, as I had already splinted his left arm and sutured some lacerations. I was aware that he was also under the influence of drugs. One of the ER workers did something to him that he didn't like or perhaps made him uncomfortable, maybe an adjustment of the splint. I was standing on his right side and saw his right hand go to his right front pants pocket. He grabbed onto something in that front pocket, and when he pulled the object out with thumb and index finger, it was the biggest handgun that I have ever seen—and it looked especially huge at that close distance. I instinctively wrestled the gun from him before he could get his hand around it, and I threw it over on the counter behind me. A loose gun in the ER gets lots of attention, so we had plenty of help immediately— and the police got to come back. I guess we assumed that they had searched him during their first visit, but apparently not. I have no idea how he was able to keep that huge gun in that small front pocket of those tight jeans without it being discovered. I certainly had not seen it, and we had been all over him during his treatment. The police hadn't seen it either.

Up to this point, I've written what I can easily remember. In 1984 I began using a Week at a Glance log books, which I kept up with ever since, and the following stories were jogged by those entries. I wish I had started the calendar at the beginning of general practice, as I'm sure there must be much of interest that I have forgotten. One such case was the thirteen-year-old boy who set his alarm for 2:00 a.m. so that he could get up and chop up his sister with a machete. Do ya think that was premeditated? The sister did okay, though, because she came in with only a three-centimeter laceration on her back.

An elderly gentleman arrived one day, transported by the nursing home, who said they would not take him back. They reportedly were tired of replacing Foley catheters that he had pulled out. We explained that it was fairly common behavior for patients to pull out their Foleys. They said, "No, you don't understand. He is pulling Foleys out of all the *other* patients." I don't know if the home thought we were a dumping ground for undesirables, but once the patient was in a bed, they had us. Similarly, grown children would sometimes bring their aged parents in when the children wanted to be away for a weekend. They had some crazy expectation that we would find a reason to admit both parents.

"Ronda" had fingernails eight inches long. She had been growing the ones on her right hand for ten years and the ones on the left for five years. They were not as beautiful as one would expect. The nails curved in like claws and had about a half inch of scaly, dried skin-like substance on their undersides. The patient was anorexic and had other emotional problems. She was a *former* computer operator.

I was on duty at JCL ER on Sunday, April 1, 1984. In the first two hours that morning we had a twenty-year-old brought in dead, with his head crushed in an auto accident, a forty-year-old from the same accident with fractures of several cervical vertebrae accompanied by paralysis from the nipple line down, and a grand total of five admits by 9:00 a.m.

For approximately six to twelve months in 1984, we had multiple calls to ER nurses all over town by "the glove man." He would start out by asking if the ER had rubber gloves and whether the nurse knew how to put them on. The conversation would slowly deteriorate into dirty, deviant sexual talk, all centered around rubber gloves. He would keep a new victim on the line for a considerable time and was very good at slowly escalating the filth of his talk and questions. He seemed to take pride—or joy—in how long he could drag out the call before the nurse would catch on and hang up. He was eventually caught, but I'm not sure whether he was breaking any laws. He was quite disruptive to most of the ERs in town. After a while, the nurses who were familiar with him would put him on speaker phone so that all could enjoy.

I have finished looking through the 1984 "Week at a Glance" appointment/address book. I have those books from 1984 to 2005 and hope to glean some additional stories from notes in these books. There were only five events from the 1984 book. Reading them made me sick to my stomach, though, as I remembered how busy that year was. I was offering hours to three ERs—St Luke's, JCL, and Desert Valley. That was the year I attempted to join the group at Desert Valley. We also spent considerable time talking with Bill, a financial advisor from Kansas City who flew to Phoenix several times, sometimes with a second person, to set up a financial plan for us. We knew we were not up-to-date on finances and were not taking advantage of what others were doing. We thought he could catch us up quickly. Some of his suggestions were good, but most were risky and expensive. We incorporated, which was complicated and expensive; we did a revocable family trust, which was good and we still have; and we got set up to buy insurance and we loaded investments from him on a monthly basis. Fortunately, I took the time to review the entire plan one day and stopped it. I have just now reviewed my dismissal letter to Bill from July of 1985, showing him why the plan didn't make any financial sense except for him. His split-dollar insurance plan was complicated and expensive. By incorporating, some of our money was actually taxed twice. We wanted the plan in order to make provisions for the kids' educations, and Bill's plan was for that to come "from future increase in earnings." In fairness to Bill, the plan was set up with the assumption that I would be an owner of a business and not employed, in which case the incorporation might have made more sense. I liked his ideas on tax shelters, and unfortunately, I did buy some from another source over the next few years. One of these went into bankruptcy several days after we bought it. We had invested and lost ten thousand dollars in that one, and soon after, I received a letter from the IRS that we would owe them thirty thousand because of the leverage provisions in the investment. We heard of a widow who had invested $180,000 in this one and who about had a heart attack when she received her IRS letter. We did come out almost even on the tax shelters after the big write-offs—and I assume that the widow did too—but it was complicated and scary.

I was on the St. Luke's Credentials Committee for most of my time at St. Luke's. We met monthly to review new doctor applicants to the staff and to renew current members. Not everyone who applies gets on a hospital staff, and that is some small protection to the patients who are treated there, although the screening is pretty loose. We would essentially evaluate their applications for inconsistencies, check the number and type of lawsuits the applicant had accumulated, and see if any committee members knew of any negative information about the doctor. Increasingly, doctors get sued before even getting out of their residencies. Some end up with over ten suits. Some of these are incompetent doctors, but many just have irritating personalities that draw suits. I always thought that we were giving too much credibility to lawyers and the legal system in using suits in any part of our credential screening. Doing our reviews this way is discriminatory but lends a degree of efficiency for hospitals. I believe there should be some interhospital and interstate information exchange so that any truly incompetent medical events or disciplinary actions could be considered. As a matter of fact, with the advancements in computers, one centralized database of information on each doctor could be made accessible on the national level. While this seems big-brotherish, I think federal licensing of doctors makes sense and would avoid some of the pettiness and politics at the state and local levels.

One interesting little tidbit from my 1984 Week at a Glance book is that I worked with an ER doctor who was an heir to the Brach Candy Company. Her name was Candy Brach, and I always thought that was cute. She was a good doctor and a sweet person.

On January 30, 1985, a man had gone to his doctor for a physical and was told that he had a "bad EKG." Because of this information, the man picked up his brother and both went out and got roaring drunk. After getting home at 3:00 a.m., he fell on his front steps and cut his knee. The wife awakened and told the man that while he was out drinking, his doctor had called and that the EKG result was a mistake and it was normal. I sutured the laceration, but the man said to send the bill to his doctor.

On February 1 we received an unconscious overdosed man who had been found in a front yard. He apparently had "shot up" in a lady's house, so she did what she knew to do—she filled his pants with ice and put him out in her front yard for the paramedics to pick up. Apparently, there is a street belief that ice in the shorts and around the genitalia is the preferred treatment for an overdose. We gave him Narcan, whereupon he immediately awakened and wondered where all that ice had come from.

I believe the next story was told to me. An eighty-year-old couple went to the doctor for their premarital exams. After the exams, the doctor told the man that his wife-to-be had acute angina. The man replied, "Yes, I know. I've already seen it."

I can still see another cute older couple who had come in because of a complication from the excision of a facial lesion. I asked them what the laboratory result was on the lesion. She volunteered, "Well, the autopsy showed..." Once she realized that she had said "autopsy," they both broke into laughter.

I once ran a pediatric code at St. Luke's. The parents had placed the child in its infant seat on a counter at home and it had fallen off. The infant apparently survived, at least initially, because we transferred the child to the pediatric intensive care unit at Good Sam Hospital. This was the same day that we had the "floorboard" delivery in the car, according to my notes.

I don't remember this one, but I have notes that a kid was taking hallucinogens and cut off his penis and flushed it down the stool. Maybe someone else had seen the patient and told others about the case.

An addict injected his ulnar artery once instead of a vein, resulting in severe pain with spasming of the artery and loss of blood supply to the area it supplies. I've recorded another incident of an old female druggie who pinched my butt as she walked down the aisle behind where we were writing on charts. The nurses observed the action and wouldn't let me live it down. Another old lady who didn't like me requested that I get her an "older doctor." I informed her that I was the oldest doctor in the building—and probably the *only* doctor in the building at that time of night. Another 104-year-old lady stated cutely, "I thought I was old when I was 103."

It was a usual messy, miserable Saturday evening in the St. Luke's ER. The rooms were full and, as usual, there was not enough nursing help to keep up with the patient volume. An ambulance rolled in bringing an old lady with gastrointestinal complaints. She was "vomiting up her toes," and it would not have been appropriate for her to stay on the gurney in the entryway. Another less miserable patient was moved out of the trauma room and this lady was placed in there on the ER cot. The old lady was so miserable that she kept her head and face covered with a large towel while she continued to upchuck into a small basin that was grossly inadequate for the job.

A pleasant young man came to the front desk and asked to be with his mother, so he was hastily shown into the room by the secretary. I had seen that vomiting lady early-on by myself and had ordered diagnostic studies and an IV, which were started. We just did not have enough nurses to give adequate care and comfort to someone so ill. Because of this and the fact that he was just a good caring person, the young man gave most of her personal care himself. He repeatedly emptied that basin full of vomit as she would hand it out from under the towel. He supported her head as best he could and held her hand during much of the stay. The smells were bad, and the vomit on his hands and clothing was extremely unpleasant. It doesn't seem to bother one so much when it's your own mother. At some point, a nurse came into the room to obtain vitals, which necessitated removal of the towel from the lady's face. Their eyes met for the first time and I don't know who was the most surprised. The man yelled, "You're not my mother!" and the lady whimpered, "You're not my son." I hope in retrospect the man could have some kind of good feeling about helping a stranger.

Chapter Eleven

Transitions

1996–2001

Thomas-Davis Clinics offered me a position in their urgent care facilities in 1996 that appeared too good to pass up. They were the largest of the HMO clinics in Phoenix and seemed stable. It was a chance to have daytime hours and a lower acuity. For the first time, I totally retired from St. Luke's. Thomas-Davis had a non-compete clause in the contract that would not allow one to work anywhere else while employed by them. As an HMO provider, this new experience seemed to be the coming thing in medicine. They contracted with state agencies and employers to provide affordable care to their employees. This was called managed care and was accomplished by employing doctors for basic care and contracting with only a few specialists.

Problems with this system were immediately apparent to everyone. The specialists were either employed or contracted at such a low rate that they had no reason to be appreciative of our referrals. Now when we called them, they may have already been paid for work we were asking them to do. The employed primary care doctors had no incentive to see large numbers of patients, especially late in the day. There was nothing to prevent them from sending any latecomers to urgent care—and I wonder what kept them from just sending *everything* there. Some of them saw twelve patients per day and called that a heavy load, whereas many doctors see double that number.

We had mandatory weekly meetings for all of the Thomas Davis doctors in Phoenix in which quality of care was discussed. It was hard to disguise the real sense of the meeting, which was how we could give quality care for less money. I felt sorry for the administrative staff who had to ride that fine line. I respect them for trying, as this focus was a new concept in medicine. HMOs still exist, so someone must have cured some of the early concerns.

The urgent-care setting provided fewer interesting cases. One day, a mother brought in her two-year-old daughter with a sore throat. When she saw the condition of her child's throat with my light, she nearly fainted. The throat and soft palate were blood red and obviously traumatized. The mother broke down and said she suspected abuse, and then all kinds of government agencies got involved. I never had to testify, so someone must have thoroughly confessed. In another event, our twenty-something security guard shot and killed himself. Somewhere around that time, a city worker committed suicide by jumping head first into one of those huge tree choppers on the corner near the urgent care office.

Thomas-Davis was purchased by five DOs from California, and I thought, *uh-oh*. I had just been through changes of ownership several times at other hospitals, which usually resulted in changes that were worse for us. They tried to reduce our incomes while presenting the changes as positives for us. The doctors at Thomas-Davis were unhappy with the double-talk, and I decided to leave in September of 1997 to go to work at West Valley Emergicenter and Wickenburg ER. My malpractice tail, about $12,000, was paid by Thomas-Davis. Malpractice "tail" is the part of malpractice insurance that would cover suits that might be filed after leaving a job. The whole Thomas-Davis system went belly-up a few months later, and many of the doctors who stayed until the end did not get the malpractice tail paid and had to buy it themselves.

When the bankruptcy occurred, it appeared that everyone just left. The urgent-care area on the front main floor of the Thunderbird Thomas-Davis building was purchased by a friend of mine, Dr. Leyva, and he continued to run it as a private business. Except for this urgent-care area, the entire building was open and unguarded. About a month after the bankruptcy, I went upstairs and got my employee files (which were interesting) and my picture. It was spooky. Everything was in place except for the people. That such a busy place now appeared as though everyone had just "up and left" with no concern for patient files and apparently no arrangements for continuation of patient care, was strange. There was no money to pay for termination of the business. Nothing is forever, and it is good to remember that any documents are potentially wide open in a business that either closes suddenly or is under subpoena.

I left Thomas-Davis on September 1, 1997, which was the exact time of our move to Sun City Grand, on the west side. I had arranged for job continuity long before terminating the Thomas-Davis job, so I started full time at West Valley Emergicenter on September 2. I also did fairly heavy part time work at Wickenburg ER. Both of these were an easy drive from our new home. I must have had an unfounded fear of being without work, and thus almost always held two jobs at once.

The West Valley Emergicenter was my worst work experience ever, and I still have an unpleasant feeling when traveling anywhere near that facility. I had some basic differences with the director regarding how quickly we should see patients and the amount of documentation necessary for the visits. To be fair, they moved into a much-needed new facility during my time there, and the system was still raw. Plus, the volume exploded after the move—as happens at first with any move. This was advertised as a true emergency room, but it was not attached to a hospital. It was thought of as having a thirteen-mile-long corridor to Maryvale Samaritan Hospital, which was the sponsoring hospital. The facility accepted ambulances and high-acuity patients. A radiologist was not on site twenty-four hours a day, there was no one to call for help, and doctors seldom came to the facility to see their patients—or for consults. All admits went to the hospital by ambulance or helicopter. We were thus responsible for giving critical care to those awaiting transport to the hospital. This could easily tie up most of our nursing staff. I vividly remember one time having four MI (myocardial infarction) patients in the area near the ambulance doors, awaiting transport. I had worked in fully 25 percent of the emergency rooms in Phoenix by that time and felt I knew what the standard of care should be. Doctors who work in a system like that develop coping mechanisms and shortcuts to be able to tolerate what they do. Unfortunately, business decisions and higher hourly incomes often drive what happens. I have always thought a true ER should have times of being less busy so they can handle the inevitable surges of patients. We now have a crisis in which ERs are fully busy all the time, so when the surges come, something has to give. That "give" can mean decreased quality of care and longer patient wait times.

An interesting sidelight to the West Valley experience was how administrative ideas can impact patient care and the atmosphere that exists. Someone thought it would be nice to have a $50,000 grand piano in the waiting room of the new facility at West Valley. No one played it and no one could touch it, but we had a piano. It appeared to me like an expensive façade on an old building, or chrome wheels on a junker car. Some philanthropist probably donated the piano specifically for that location, in which case it wouldn't make sense to not take it. It just seemed silly, given the need for better patient care in many crucial areas. Several ERs tried to provide the smell of homemade bread in the air by actually baking bread. Food smells don't mix well with the usual ER smells, and many found them nauseating rather than pleasant. In several instances, an ER would have some expensive, showy piece of equipment that none of us could operate or would ever need, but which would look good and be pointed out on tours of the facility.

From the first of November 1997 thru September of 1999, I did full- or part-time work at Wickenburg, always supplemented by John C. Lincoln, which was my "old faithful" and my only work from September 1999 until retirement in 2001.

The nearly two years at Wickenburg were pleasant. The facility was a nice thirty-minute drive from our SCG home to the hospital. We could work twenty-four-hour shifts, so travel was not a big issue. These small-town people were rugged, some ranchers, and very nice. The town has been known for producing some of the best cowboys in the world and several world-famous (and expensive) treatment centers for addictions and bulimia. The hospital had about eighteen beds and was old, but well kept. We had a full-time lab with x-ray on call, but a radiologist was only there in the mornings during the week. Like most small-town hospitals, anything that really *needs* to be admitted is not admitted locally. The doctors fear the patient's condition will deteriorate, and then transfer might not be appropriate or even possible. If there are doctors within transport distance better qualified to care for that condition (and there usually are), it is too risky to keep them under local care. One can just hear the lawyers ask, "Doctor, did you really think you, a primary-care physician, could better care for this patient than the super specialist just thirty miles away?" This is one of the reasons I left general practice.

For the above reasons, there are many transfers to the city from small-town ERs. The next question that presents is mode of transfer. Too frequently, an expensive helicopter transport takes place rather than transporting via ambulance. If something goes wrong in the ambulance transfer, the ER doctor is on the hook. Again, you can hear the lawyers say, "Mr. ER doctor, helicopter transfer was readily available. Did you not think this patient deserved the more rapid means of transfer?" A helicopter ride may be three- to four-thousand dollars versus an ambulance ride in the few hundreds. God forbid the patient in question had been poor, as that would just give the lawyer more ammunition to make the doctor appear uncaring or even negligent in choosing the less expensive means of transport.

Government regulations can also affect transportation decisions by forcing the patient to be kept locally. These regulations were introduced to prevent the "dumping" of non-paying patients on other hospitals. The dumping was usually carried out upon county hospitals, when we had them. The county hospitals now say they are "private," but they are still good at finding government money to care for the poor—but that's another subject. The anti-dumping regulations say that one hospital cannot transfer to another facility if the original hospital has the ability to care for that patient. An appropriate transfer required phone contact, requesting the second facility accept the patient, and paperwork documenting these actions on both ends had to be completed. The real reason for this was to keep the nicer, private hospitals from being selective with their patients, particularly in regard to paying versus nonpaying patients. Another aspect of this is that now, anyone who appears at the ER door has to be evaluated. The next patient to appear at the door could be the hospital's million-dollar-loss case. Hospitals are responsible to care for that patient until he either gets better, dies, or can be transferred. A high percentage of ER patients, over 50 percent in some areas, either cannot—or will not—pay their bills. I still don't understand how hospitals can afford to have an emergency department, given the above risks. Maybe it comes from the ten-dollar aspirin that the rest of us are charged. Those of us who are dumb enough to work for a living are paying for the care given to the rest, anyway. Seems like a good argument for government-run medicine.

One other point, and then I will get off this boring subject. The feds have added some real teeth to their non-funded initiative here. They implemented a $50,000 fine against any physician who performed an inappropriate transfer, plus the same fine against the hospital from which the transfer occurred. I believe it is even higher now. The federal regulators, of course, judge this retrospectively. It is illegal to buy insurance to cover this fine. These rulings fan the original fear that we discussed—that of a physician admitting someone we shouldn't. Do you keep a case, and risk being sued? Or do you transfer the patient and risk being fined for an inappropriate transfer? That is, if you can even talk someone into accepting the transfer.

Wickenburg was a good place to work, but the facility did share some of the above stresses—as would any small-town emergency department. The hospital changed ER groups three times while I was there, and it was finally purchased by a large hospital group from out of state. I had been through this before. They replaced many of the locals, who knew how to make the place run, with temporary help at three times the cost. My decision to move on, though, was made when one day I noticed, from behind, three donut-eating, meeting-loving, pear-shaped, briefcase-carrying home office folks walking three abreast, totally filling the hospital corridor. They were there to *help* us. To be fair, they did infuse lots of money into the facility, and some of it probably did some good.

The local people working at the Wickenburg hospital were very nice, as are most small-town folk. My day book shows that I worked there until September 1999.

I had been doing heavy part-time work at John C. Lincoln (JCL) ER, and at that time they stepped up my hours to essentially full time until I retired August 1, 2001. The hospital had developed an after-hours and weekend urgent-care area out of a room close to the ER, and most of my remaining work time was spent there. The Lincoln group had always been good to me, and this arrangement allowed me to finish my work days with lower stress.

.

Chapter Twelve

Retirement

August 1, 2001–Present

My 2001 "Week at a Glance" book says that my last work day was at Lincoln on July 29, 2001. We stayed busy with travels to the Midwest during the remainder of 2001. Twyla flew back to Iowa to see her folks three times, and we drove back twice. We attended an Otte reunion on one of those trips in August. For several years, we spent from one to three months back home in Clarinda, Iowa, each summer, trying to make it possible for Twyla's folks to stay in their home. Mervil died in 2005, and the house was adapted so Mabel could stay alone. She broke a hip on July 4, 2005, and after that she was unable to stay alone. Mabel died in 2007.

Our home and lot are smaller than what we had in Scottsdale. It is easier to care for and can be closed up easier for trips. We enjoy the grass and trees around our property, and also the fact that we don't have to take care of it. Our children enjoy the home and seem to like coming here.

The activities and facilities at Sun City Grand (SCG) are tremendous. We haven't utilized the facilities as much as we had expected, nor as much as others do. Our activities are centered around family and out-of-state visitors. I spend considerable time on the computer, doing research and managing investments. Finishing this book is a priority, but it keeps getting put off. Twyla continues to do much volunteer work with the Phoenix Art Museum.

Twyla's sister Carolyn and husband Doug Drake moved to SCG soon after we did. They had been looking at the Sun Cities for some time also. They have a home four miles away and are here at SCG about seven months of the year and in Des Moines for the summers. Their local social life is more active here than ours, and they play lots of golf, so we don't see them very much.

Some of our Clarinda relatives and friends have started renting homes in SCG for some of the winter months. They can use all of the facilities during their rental time. They really enjoy the amenities here, especially the four great golf courses. My sister Irma and her husband Larry have done this every year and have now bought a house here. We get to see them and their friends, so their vacation becomes ours. Our children all enjoy coming over and don't want us to move.

My citrus orchard is limited by space at the SCG home, but I have managed to squeeze in eleven trees, mostly dwarf varieties. I have tried very hard to have a garden, now that I have time for that. Rabbits and birds eat everything here, though, so I have had to abandon the garden idea. There are lots of coyotes in the area that do not appear at all afraid of humans. One came within two feet of our kitchen window in the area between the casita and the house. They still don't keep the rabbits under control—maybe they are sick of rabbit fur. I believe they eat some of the plants too.

Three of our children (Valerie, Pam, and Pat and their families) moved back to Arizona during this time and lived about three miles north of the Scottsdale home where they had lived since 1980, through their high school and college years. I should also mention that we had eleven grandchildren during those eight years and six of them live about forty-five minutes away. Kim and family moved from Minneapolis to Rochester, Minnesota, during that time frame. Pam and Phil and their family have since moved to the Denver area.

People from Phoenix don't seem to understand or care about the difference in the Sun Cities. Most of those who move here are from out of state, and few are transplants from within the Phoenix metropolitan area. The original Sun City contained about forty thousand homes and was started about fifty years ago. Sun City West was built later and had about twenty thousand homes. Sun City Grand is about twenty years old now and has about ten thousand homes. Since no children were allowed, the original Sun City and most of Sun City West paid no taxes to support schools. That did not go over well with the rest of the community, and I have to agree that it was not fair. That has since changed, and we pay full school taxes. There are lots of local jokes about "Sun City people." I will give some of my observations later, but then I may have to leave town.

Del Webb was good at what he did, and he and his wife have been doing it for a long time. I am told that he did some work for "the mob" in Las Vegas and built The Flamingo. He built his retirement facilities first, with exercise rooms, pools, and extensive meeting areas. The homes came afterward. Many of the homes were built to line the golf courses, and those courses would have been in use before the homes were built around them. He built many first-class exercise and community centers so no one would be very far from facilities. He had learned what would work and what wouldn't, so would not let buyers make stupid mistakes. The yards grew smaller so he could pack more homes into the later developments and charge a hefty premium for golf course lots. We paid an extra $65,000 for our lot, but I have heard that some homes on the golf course now go for $200,000 extra. One could buy homes without the extra fee and would have everything except the golf course views. Sun City Grand residents now pay over $1,370 per year per home for association dues, but for that they have the use of two beautiful recreation facilities which feature five heated pools, an indoor running track, great weight machines, courts for nearly any game you want, hobby shops, a ball diamond, meeting rooms, and entertainment facilities. The yearly assessment also covers the beautiful plantings in the common areas and entrances. The fee is per home and is practically guaranteed to go up each year. The four golf courses and the community center buildings were built by Del

Webb and have been turned over to the community association. The golf courses have been planned to be self-supporting and are among the most beautiful in the city. They are open to the public at this point, but there is significantly lower charge to residents and their guests. Three of them could be closed to the public if resident use warrants it. Pulte bought Del Webb several years ago, and I suspect this may not be a positive, but most of the above plans were in place.

The Del Webb business plan was such that folks would come to look, be overwhelmed, and buy. The details could be completed easily from their out-of-state home. Twyla and I, on the other hand, must have driven them nuts, as we lived in nearby Scottsdale and came over frequently. We were looking at Sun City West one day when Zelpha, our sales person, mentioned that their newest development, Sun City Grand, was being planned. She told us how to get there, so we went down R. H. Johnson and across Grand to a graded-up road where Sunrise Road would eventually be. The road had been graded up quite high and had no smoothed surface, but our van made it quite a ways, until we were stopped by security. They informed us that the development was not yet open to the public, but that we were welcome to come back when it opened, which we did.

Once Sun City Grand opened, we were there often. We lived in Scottsdale and traveled over frequently, obsessing over each decision. We spent considerable time picking our lot, home, inside options, and landscaping. We purchased all of this from Del Webb even though their extras were more expensive, justifying the expense because I was still working. Many folks would purchase the cheapest Del Webb options and then would rip them out and put in better quality upgrades from local vendors.

We fought for the changes we wanted. Often the things we asked for would not be available, only to become so before we closed. We had 130 changes in our home, which Zelpha said was a record. At one time she even said "Carl, you can't have everything." Because we had just been through the buying process, we at one time considered purchasing an additional home as an investment. It would have taken only a single day of work, and in retrospect, would have been a good thing. We did get the full three-car garage and the four-foot extension on our main garage. We were so tired of easing ourselves out of the cars many times per day in our previous homes because the garage was too small. The thing that we did not get was more room in the utility room, which is still a bottleneck for entering and carrying groceries into the house. I do enjoy my large garage, and it has proven to be a source of joy. We did an epoxy coating on the floor, which allows me to scrub the floor to a shine. This annoys the neighbor men to no end, as their wives now expect them to keep a similar garage. Bob once said, "Carl, it's just a garage."

It seems there are always homes for sale here. The turnover rate for the Sun Cities is about seven percent per year, while the rate for the entire city is about five percent. We frequently hear sirens around 7:00 each morning, and I tell Twyla, "Someone *else* didn't wake up." She especially dislikes my imitation going something like this: "Henry honey, time to get up. Henry, *Henry*—aargh!" When golfers hear sirens they just say, "Another golf cart available."

Seeing the dance classes or interest groups dancing away in the middle of a hot day is somewhat surreal. A columnist was at one of these dances when a dancer collapsed and died. He noted that the paramedics came and did their thing, but that the dancing continued uninterrupted.

Old people do strange things. If there is a line, they will get in it and wait forever. Don't ever cut in front of one or leave too much room between you and the one ahead. They like to be right on your tail and expect you to do the same to the one ahead. They seem to think they need to stop their cars completely before turning off a busy road, as if they think their car will overturn if they take the corner too fast. They seem to not know where the brake is, but they do apply the horn long before they think of breaking. We always feel very threatened while driving in Sun City West and have had many close calls. Word to the wise: ignore turn signals.

I once saw an old lady push the "walk" button at an intersection and then proceed immediately across eight lanes of Bell Road, apparently thinking that pushing that button allowed her to proceed immediately. The most common conversation heard when residents exit a building is, "Now where the hell did we park?"

Old people are always early, and the saying here is that if you are on time, you are late. The elderly love to save seats for their friends, and they don't mind asking you to help. Get behind one in a grocery store, and you might as well take another aisle. They seem to have no clue what is behind them, and it is almost impossible to get their attention or pass them. If you leave a reasonable distance ahead of you in line, they will cut in and act like they don't see you. This has happened to me the last three times at the pharmacy. We are requested to stay back a reasonable distance for the privacy of the person at the counter. An old person or couple will slither in, ignore the line, and appear oblivious to any amount of grunting or attempts to get their attention. They will complete their business and never look anyone in the eye. Farts are common, and there is just nothing else that sounds like a fart. We try to avoid the senior discount days at the stores. Many seniors will argue with the poor clerk over a discount of only a few cents, oblivious of the long line waiting behind them.

Driving into Sun City Grand any time after 8:00 p.m. would cause one to wonder if the community had been the victim of a dirty bomb attack, where all the people have been killed and property left unscathed. When coming home in the late evening, I have often said, "They're all dead!" People arise early but retire early. Some areas have very little front lighting, which adds to the feeling that the community has been abandoned. I believe most are just too tight financially to light the fronts of their houses. Some of the tightest millionaires in the world live here. Seven of the eight on our cul-de-sac are millionaires—and I'm not sure about the eighth.

Despite the fun I make of us, these are the types of folks who won World War II. They have been in middle management and worked hard for their money. Good value for their money is what brings them here. The filthy rich go elsewhere.

The golf courses have signs all over saying that the golfer is responsible for any damage to homes or private property. We have had three broken windows and multiple pock marks on the house from golf balls. No golfer has ever come forward to take responsibility or see if we were okay. We have always paid for the window and house repairs ourselves. We had our back patio door open recently and a nice man hit a ball that ended up inside our house through the open screen door. The ball hit one of our guests in the leg as he sat at our dining table. Another time, one of the grandchildren was having a crying fit as his parents were departing. I went to close the patio door and noted the man standing on the knoll by our patio, looking our way, with a genuinely concerned look on his face. He was worried that his ball had hit a child. I felt bad for him, as it took me a little while to realize what his concern was and to alleviate his fears, and I threw his ball back to him.

There have been several of what I call "Clara-isms" during this time frame. I was helping Twyla babysit at the Mersiowskys when Clara was two or three years old. The bibs that they use are the kind that have to be snapped together to form the pocket to catch food. I tried to snap Clara's bib, but had not done that type before and was having trouble getting the bib constructed properly. Clara finally grabbed the bib away from me and held it toward Grandma and said, "Here, Grandma, you do this. Grandpa is a slow learner."

Another "Clara" episode took place at one of the holidays at our Sun City Grand home at about the same time. All four of our children, their spouses, and our eleven grandchildren attended for the opportunity to be together and experience one of Grandma Twyla's meals. People often do their own thing, and I was taking a shower. Clara wandered into our bedroom and saw me in the mirror getting out of the shower. She promptly went back to the rest of the guests in the living room and announced, "Grandpa has a saggy butt."

We have a total of eleven grandchildren. Valerie and Pat still live in Scottsdale; Pam in Denver (Highland's Ranch); and Kim in Rochester, Minnesota. We still like life in Sun City Grand, but we travel to the kids' homes frequently. Larry and Irma visited here, staying from one to three months each winter, and they recently bought a beautiful home in Sun City Grand. Four of their Iowa friends have purchased winter homes here in Sun City Grand as well. I am eighty-two years old and Twyla is seventy-nine, so our next move will probably be closer to some of the kids and to some unit that can give us more care. Nothing much funny has happened in the past few years, but a couple of stories from our years here are probably worth telling.

Sal was an Italian and a good sport. He lived at the entrance of our cul-de-sac and loved to be teased—even though he would loudly complain about it. He was a strong Democrat, so Republican bumper stickers kept appearing on his car—as well as a tailpipe whistle and fake bullet holes and scratches. I didn't realize Sal didn't know about the bugs in Iowa called democrats. He took real offense one time when we came back from the Midwest and talked of killing democrats in Iowa. One time, he planted a new citrus tree in his front yard, and I went over that night and tied all manner of other fruits on his tree. He was truly confused to see bananas and apples on his new tree the next morning. He told everyone about his new tree.

Sal was a little overweight but lost forty pounds over a period of a few months. I assumed that he had a cancer, but nothing was found. Some of his family came to live with him for a month and determined that he had Alzheimer's and was simply forgetting to eat. He was moved to a facility in California to be near his family. I called this Italian several months later and asked him how he liked it at the new home. Sal, true to his usual self, said, "Great! Lots of women, lots of women."

It's a little discouraging, but at least five from our cul-de-sac have had to be moved back to other parts of the country to be near their families due to Alzheimer's or dementia. The saddest and most challenging aspect is that most will reject their diagnosis and will use all their coping mechanisms to appear normal. Some become very angry at even a hint of the diagnosis and any restriction of their activity. Sometimes it takes a while before the families become involved.

In those first years, we had block parties about every three months. We never knew whether Sal would come or whether he would boycott the party. Following is a letter that I sent to Sal in 2002—a time when we were all younger and having more fun.

September 18, 2002

Mr. Sal Giammona

20118 North Lagos Court

Surprise, AZ 85374

Dear Mr. Giammona:

It has been brought to our attention, thru some of your neighbors, that your house and the one directly to your left have been produced with exactly the same color scheme—and, in fact, have the same roof tile colors. There was apparently a fuch up when laying out The Desert Bloom Division, which caused this anomaly to occur involving lots 145 and 146. This is in direct contradistinction to the CCR's for your area, so the color scheme on one of the houses must be changed.

In order to be completely fair and impartial about the resolution of this problem, our secretaries drew straws for both homeowners. Congratulations!!!! You came up with the short straw and will receive a new paint and tile job. We feel that this will solve the problem to everyone's satisfaction. The new look will be entirely free to you and will make your home unlike your neighbors—in fact, unlike any of your neighbors.

Our paint crew will be at your house early on Monday, September 23 to begin the conversion. The color scheme that our retro-designers has selected has the following:

Main stucco color: Bright Green

Wood trim: Dark Purple

Roof tile: Black

Please remove your car from the garage on that morning and park it at the end of the cul-de-sac for safety. It will also be necessary for you to empty the garage so that we may carry the new color design to all areas that can be seen from the street.

Thank you in advance for your cooperation in this and again, CONGRATULATIONS.

Sincerely,

_____

Will Pullteeth, Director

Color Coordination Community Controller, Pulte/Webb

Sun City Grand

For some reason, I thought it would also be funny to send the following letter to all the neighbors on our cul-de-sac in 2006. You have to understand that the far end of our street overlooks the driving range of Desert Springs. The letter that follows was distributed, and by 9:00 that same evening I realized it was too real and that the SCG board and lawyers were soon going to be involved—probably by morning. So I made late night visits to those neighbors to inform them that this was only a joke. I almost failed to convince some of them to refrain from taking action.

Surprise, Arizona

November 11, 2006

Webb/Pulte Public Relations Department

Sun City Grand

Arizona

Dear Lagos Court Resident:

We are contacting all of the residents of your cul-de-sac to inform you of some changes being planned for your area. You have probably noticed the marks on the asphalt near the end of your street. We allowed it to be thought, initially, that these marks were the result of the Otte grandchildren playing with sidewalk chalk. Our project is now far enough along that we need to inform you that these are utility company markings. These are only the first of many more markings which will extend up the rest of Lagos Court and be followed by extensive utility excavations in the street. This project is expected to continue for at least one year. Since you will not be able to utilize your garages, we have arranged to allow your parking on both sides of Starlight Drive, anywhere within three blocks of its intersection with Lagos.

The project that we mentioned is Desert Springs Driving Range Manor. The driving range will be closed on January 1 and we have elected to exercise our right to convert this area to homes. There will be 106 very attractive patio type homes built within the area now occupied by the driving range. Lagos Court will be extended down into this development and will be the only access to and from these homes.

We beg your forbearance during this build-out and do realize that it will make your street much busier than that to which you are accustomed. We thank you for your understanding of our need to make these changes.

Sincerely,

_____

Max Outofluck

Webb/Pulte Public Relations Division

Sun City Grand, Arizona

Following is another letter intended to be a joke to my neighbors on Lagos Court. These are distributed when something happens in the community or appears that might raise concern to those who worry too much.

October 12, 2017

Dear Lagos Court Resident:

As a North Lagos Court Resident, you have probably noticed the porta potty and construction activity near the house on the corner, previously owned by Jim and Ginny Lambright. It has now been sold and the current owners have given Pulte/Dell Webb some latitudes that may affect you and about which you should know.

We at the CAM office have long known that our landscape employees need a place to relieve themselves during their long workdays. For this reason, we have gained permission to place a permanent porta potty on the property at the end of your cul-de-sac. The several cement trucks seen today were providing the material to line the large underground receptacle beneath this toilet and to cement in the outhouse itself in order to make it a permanent fixture of Lagos Court.

We realize that there may be some odor from this project and we will do our best to combat that. The tank will be emptied monthly by an attractive "honey truck" and we will be experimenting with the spreading of the evacuate onto the driving range just beyond the facility.

You, living on Lagos Court, will have full access to and use of this new facility, as will all of the many walkers that use Lagos Court. We think that more walkers will detour to your area, specifically to make use of this facility—and it could become a popular meeting place for these people. Please keep an eye on this structure—and report any mischief to the building or any graffiti.

We thank you in advance for your understanding of our need for this and your help with accepting this new project. It has board and CAM approval—and there may be more such buildings if this proves as successful as we think it will.

Sincerely,

_____

Bill Stinker

DellWebb/Pulte comfort facility coordinator.

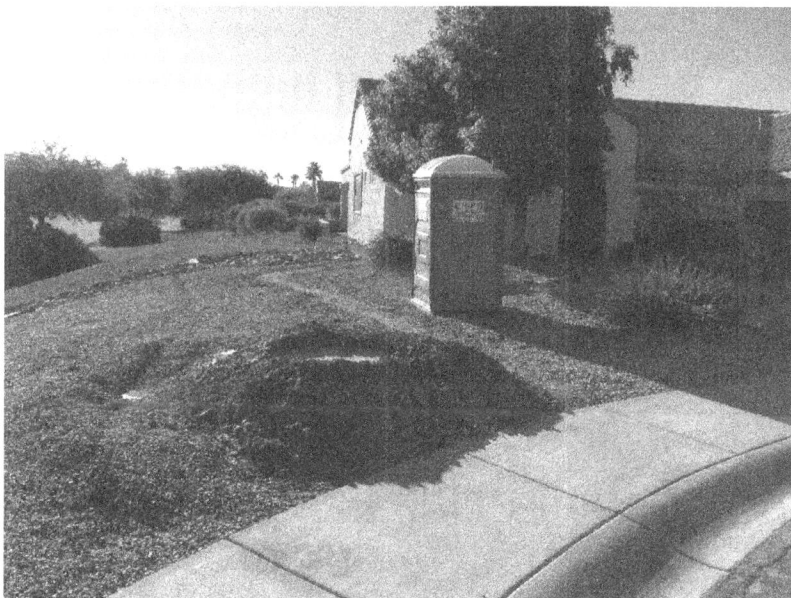

Porta Potty

I have sometimes made fun of us old people and the Sun Cities, but I do have great love and respect for them as we traverse this stage of our lives. I know also that our next move will probably be closer to some of the kids and involve more restrictive living. This has been a good step for us in our lives, and I have to recommend it. The fact that so many of our friends and relatives have bought homes is a testament to the goodness here. Imitation is the best compliment.

Thank you for reading my book.

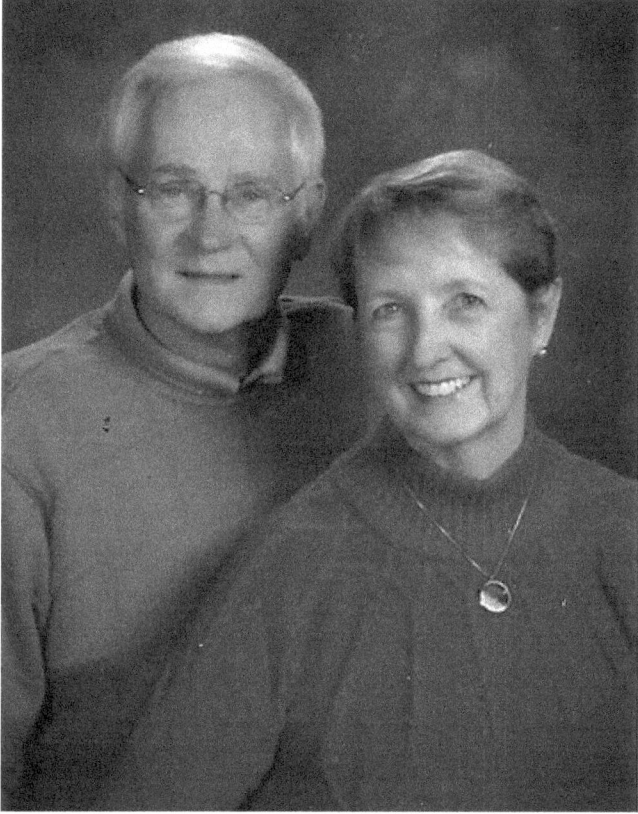

Carl and Twyla Otte

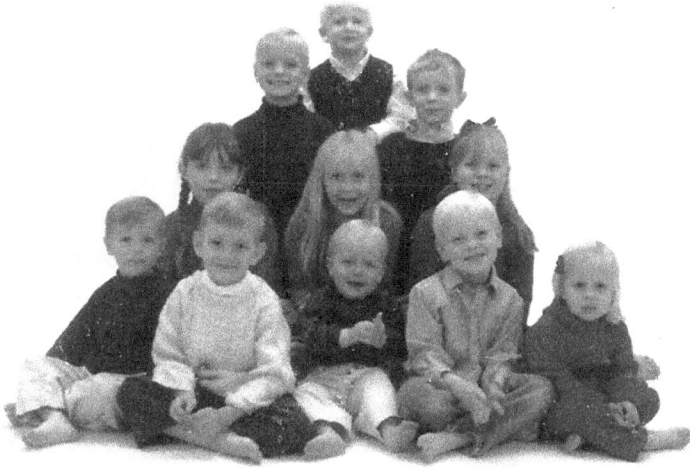

Otte Grandchildren

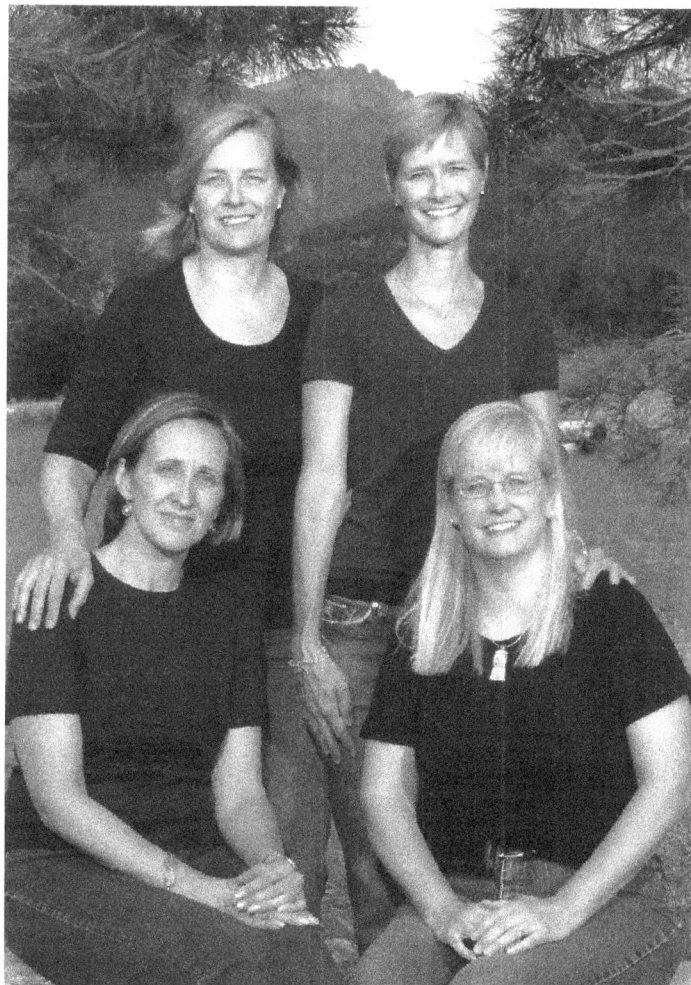

Otte Daughters
Kim, Valerie, Pam, and Pat

ABOUT THE AUTHOR

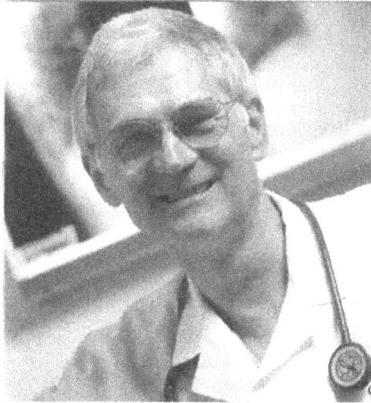

Dr. Carl Otte is an osteopathic physician who spent his first ten years in general practice in the Greeley, Colorado area. He then enrolled in one of the first emergency medicine residencies at Kansas City General Hospital, one of three graduates of the program that year. He then served two years as an air force flight surgeon at Luke Airbase in Phoenix, Arizona. He achieved board certification and practiced emergency medicine in Iowa and Arizona for fourteen more years.

Married for fifty-seven years, Dr. Otte and his wife Twyla have four daughters and eleven grandchildren.

Dr. Otte sees and remembers comedy in everyday life, but especially from his ER experiences. The ER stories must be told and preserved, and that was the impetus for starting this book. Much comedy could be found, however, in growing up on a farm and later raising one wife and four daughters—and so this book was expanded.

www.ingramcontent.com/pod-product-compliance
Lightning Source LLC
Chambersburg PA
CBHW060005210326
41520CB00009B/826